Diabetic Cookbook

Easy & Delicious Recipes for Prediabetes, Diabetes,
and Type 2 Diabetes Newly Diagnosed

WILLARD MARSH

Contents

Introduction 1

Breakfast Recipes 3

   Cinnamon and Apple Pancakes 4

   Avocado Meyer Lemon Toast 6

   Low-Carb Breakfast Spinach Smoothie 7

   Breakfast Mushroom Surprise 8

   Breakfast Barley Porridge 9

   Cheddar Breakfast Muffins 10

   English Breakfast Scones 12

   Tasty Breakfast Egg Wraps 14

   Quinoa Berry Breakfast 15

   Pepper Fajitas and Marinated Steak 16

   Diabetic Two Minutes Breakfast Smoothie 18

   Delicious Breakfast Burrito 19

   Oat, Almond, And Raspberry Breakfast Cookies 20

   Low-Carb Healthy Breakfast Smoothie 21

   Breakfast Apple Muffins Diabetic-Friendly 22

   Coconut Banana and Blueberry Porridge 23

   Breakfast Omega Seed Starter 24

   Fruity Nutty Breakfast Yogurt 25

   Spinach with Poached Eggs 26

   Kale and Pineapple Breakfast Smoothie 27

Dip Recipes 28

   Tasty Cranberry Sauce 29

   Mexican-Style Tomato Salsa 30

Peanut Satay Dip 31

Harissa and Black-Eyed Bean Dip 32

Tasty Homemade Hummus Dip 33

Simple Pea Dip 34

Simple Mint Yogurt Dip 35

Greek-Style Aubergine Dip 36

Delicious Ranch Dip 38

Tasty Dill Dip 39

Vegetarian Recipes **40**

Tasty Veggie Shepherd's Pie 41

Simple Grilled Aubergine 43

Halloumi and Quinoa Salad 44

Leek and Sun Roasted Tomatoes Frittata 45

Carrot and Chickpea Stew 46

Miso and Mushroom Broth 48

Winter Chili Vegetable 50

Delicious Okra Curry 52

Stir Fry Tangy Quorn 54

Sweet & Sour Tofu 55

Delicious Chickpea Curry 56

Tasty Vegetable mince 58

Tempting Mutter Paneer 59

Tasty Kidney Bean Curry 61

Falafel Burgers with Pita Bread 62

Spaghetti Bolognese Low-Carb 63

Tasty Vegetable Curry 65

Courgette Cheesy Frittata 66

Cashew Vegetable Stir Fry 69

Appetizer And Snacks Recipes **70**

Cream Cheese and Smoked Salmon Vol au vents 71

Tofu and Vegetable Wontons 72

Witches' Broomsticks Snack 74

Tasty Granola Bars 75

Feta Spinach Rolls 76

Scary Strawberry Snacks 78

Cabbage and Chicken Wontons 79

Easy Severed Fingers 82

Tasty Eggplant Rolls Roasted 83

Melon and Parma Ham Balls 85

Delicious Buffalo Chicken 86

Festive Pesto Mini Chicken Kebabs 87

Tempting Salmon Seaweed Wraps 88

Cocktail Nuts with Maple Glazed 90

Pigs Wrapped in Blankets 91

Delicious Watercress with Pancetta 92

Greek-Style Shrimps 93

Tasty Baba Ghanoush Eggplant Dip 94

Delicious Cheesy Polenta with Mushrooms 96

Soups And Stews Recipes **97**

Tasty Thai Green Soup 98

Tofu Soup Sweet and Sour 99

Delicious Cajun Stew 100

Tasty Braised Pork Stew 102

Kidney and Black Bean Soup 103

Tempting Tomato Soup 104

Lentil Zesty Soup 106

Simple Mushroom Soup 107

Quick and Tasty White Bean Soup 109

Spinach, Chicken and Wild Rice Soup 111

Tasty Butternut Bisque 112

Moroccan Vegetable and Lentil Soup 113

Parsnip Soup Spicy 115

Festive-Style Spinach Soup 117

Yummy Butternut Squash Soup 119

Asparagus Soup Spicy 120

Thai Mixed Veg and Coconut Soup 122

Delicious Sweetcorn Soup 123

Mushroom and Chicken Soup 125

Most Popular Diabetic Recipes 126

Toothsome Cauliflower Pizza 127

Stuffed Bell Peppers with Turkey 129

Tasty Corn on the Cob with Citrus Buttery Spread 131

Spiced Pineapple, Halibut and Pepper Skewers 132

Scrumptious Tuna Cakes with Creamy Cucumber Dipping 134

Mouth-Watering Chicken Cutlets 136

Tasty Salmon Sandwiches with Apricot Sauce 137

Grilled Peaches Topped with Cream Cheese Spicy Topping 138

Tempting Salmon Croquettes 139

Tempting Mushroom Smothered Beef Patties 141

Soy-Ginger Flavored Steak Bites 142

Steak, Chicken and Shrimp Skewers 143

Mouth-Watering Beef Chimichangas 145

Appetizing Sirloin Steak Antipasto Salad 146

Cheddar and Asparagus Chicken Breasts 147

Tasty Polenta Triangles 149

Oatmeal and Apple Cookie Crumble........................ 151

Tempting Caprese Portobello Burgers...................... 152

Toothsome Crispy Chicken Bites 153

Mediterranean-Style Turkey Burgers with Feta 154

Beef, Lamb and Pork Recipes **155**

Tempting Beef Sirloin with a Green Salad................ 156

Delicious Lamb Curry 157

Sage and Lemon Pork.. 159

Tasty Beef Teriyaki 160

Prosciutto and Tomato Panini Sandwiches................ 161

Flavorsome Spicy Beef Stew................................ 163

Pork and Plum Kebabs 164

Pork Chops Grilled with Cherry Sauce 165

Jalapenos Beef Cheeseburgers.............................. 166

Beef Stuffed Eggplants...................................... 167

Marinated Mini Beef Skewers............................... 169

Balsamic Beef, Onion and Mushrooms 170

Appetizing Lamb Shashlik 172

Balsamic Pork Chops Grilled 173

Garlic Beef Brochettes Grilled 174

Tempting Lamb Kebabs with Verdant Salsa............... 175

Caramelized Onion and Brie Burgers...................... 177

Tasty Lamb Meatballs 179

No-Cook Sweet and Sour Ham Kebabs.................... 181

Lamb Steak with a Tomato Sauce 182

Fish And Seafood Recipes................................ **183**

COD with Spinach and Garlic 184

Tasty Chili Prawns 185

Trout Fish with Beans 186

Roasted Whole Lemon Sole with Celeriac............................ 187

BBQ Shrimps with Tropical Rice.. 188

Salmon with Cranberry Chutney Glazed............................. 190

Prawn and Avocado Cocktails... 191

Peppery Flavor COD with Mixed Veggies 192

Grilled Basil Flavor Shrimps... 193

Tasty Salmon with Basil Sauce 194

Tamarind Flavor Prawns 195

Tasty COD with Sautéed Kale 197

Easy and Quick Salmon & Tomato Twangs 199

Prawn Salad with Asparagus... 200

Flavorsome Zingy Whole Mackerel.................................... 201

Crab, Artichoke and Spinach Dip....................................... 202

Southern-Style Crab Cakes with Dipping Sauce 203

Tasty Thai-Style Fennel Tuna 205

Classic Fish Pie 207

Delicious COD Parsley Parcels 209

Chicken And Poultry Recipes **211**

Grilled Chicken with Black Beans and Corn Salsa 212

Tasty Grilled South of the Border Chicken 214

Simple and Quick Lemon Chicken...................................... 215

Crispy Chicken Nuggets with BBQ Dipping Sauce............. 216

Roasted Chopped Chicken Salad... 218

Chicken with Artichokes and Spinach 220

Chicken Salad with Spinach.. 221

Pepper-Lemon Chicken Wings.. 222

Fajita Flavor Grilled Chicken 223

Dinner Chicken Salad with a Green Onion Dressing 224

Chicken Kiev's Stuffed with Feta and Spinach 226

Tempting Sticky Chicken 228

Chicken Mushroom and Cashew Nut Risotto 229

Thai-Style Chicken Satay 231

Tasty Chicken with Asparagus 233

Thai-Style Green Chicken Curry 234

Simple Fried Chicken 236

Sizzler Chicken Wings 237

Easy and Tasty Chicken Burgers 238

Dessert Recipes **239**

Cheese and Cashew Flapjacks 240

Raspberry and Raw Apple Tart 241

Mouth-Watering Ricotta Cheesecake 242

Tasty Fruit Pizza 244

Crunchy Oatcakes 245

Witches' Apples Dessert 246

Crunchy Honey Oat Cookies 247

Tasty Milk Pudding 248

Flavorful Pecan Pancakes 250

Delicious Coconut Pannacotta 252

Tasty Ginger Snaps 253

Easy Homemade Jam 255

Peachy Crumble 256

Yummy Banana Brulee 257

Dairy-Free Chocolate and Raspberry Mousse 258

Yummy Fruit Frenzy 260

Tasty Lemon Soufflé 262

Tempting Chocolate Cake 264

Yummy Kiwi Pavlova.. 266

Tasty Almond Cupcakes 268

Conclusion.. **269**

Introduction

Diabetes is a disorder in which your blood glucose level is unusually high, also referred to as blood sugar. Blood glucose, which originates from the food you eat, is your main energy source. Insulin, a pancreatic hormone, increases glucose absorption into cells for utilization as energy. Your body may create insufficient or no insulin, or it may not utilize it properly. As a result, glucose stays in your circulation & does not reach your cells.

Getting quite enough glucose in your blood can cause health problems in the long run. Even though there is exactly no cure for diabetes, you can manage it & maintain your health.

Diabetes is often known as "borderline diabetes" or "a touch of sugar." These statements indicate that someone does not have diabetes or that they have a milder type of it; yet, diabetes affects everyone.

Diabetes affected 30.3 million persons in the United States in 2015, accounting for 4% of the population. More than one-fourth of them were unaware that they had the condition. One in four adults over the age of 65 has diabetes. In adults, type 2 diabetes accounts for 90-95 percent of occurrences.

Type 1, type 2, and gestational diabetes are the three basic kinds of diabetes.

Type 1 diabetes can strike to anyone at any age, although it often strikes children and adolescents. If you have type 1 diabetes, the body generates no or very little insulin.

Adults are more likely to develop type 2 diabetes, which accounts for almost 90% of all diabetes cases. This is because your body usually does not make appropriate use of the insulin it produces when you do have type 2 diabetes. A healthy lifestyle, which includes increased physical activity and a nutritious diet, is the foundation of type 2 diabetes management.

Gestational diabetes GDM is a kind of diabetes that occurs during pregnancy and is linked to difficulties for both the mother and the child. GDM normally goes away after pregnancy, although it increases the risk of type 2 diabetes in women and their children later in life.

Breakfast Recipes

Cinnamon and Apple Pancakes

Cooking time: 20 minutes

Preparation time: 10 minutes

Servings: 8

Nutrition facts: Calories 246, Total fat 10g, Protein 5g, Carbs 33g

Ingredients:

- 2 tablespoons of agave nectar
- 200 ml of milk full-fat
- 2 medium-sized eggs
- 1/2 tablespoon of olive oil for each pancake
- 10 g of butter
- 200 g of plain flour
- 4 apples peeled, cored and sliced
- 1 teaspoon of cinnamon
- Lemon juice, to taste

Instructions:

Follow the instructions below to make cinnamon and apple pancakes.

1. In a pan melt the butter on medium for the sautéed apple.
2. Heat up for around a minute after adding the agave nectar.
3. Cook the apple slices in the mixture until they are softened. It should take approximately 10-15 minutes to complete this task.
4. Set the mixture aside after adding a spritz of lemon juice to taste.
5. For the pancakes: To create the batter, whisk the eggs well in a mixing dish before combining the flour & milk.
6. Cover the pot with a tea towel & set it aside for 10 minutes at room temperature. Cinnamon should be sprinkled over the apples that have been prepared.

7. In a small frying pan, heat 1/2 a tablespoon of olive oil.
8. Pour the mixture into the pan & tilt it to cover the entire pan's base.
9. Cook for 3 minutes on each side of the pancake, or until all sides are a light brown in color. Take out the pancake from the stove and set it aside.
10. Set the pancake on a platter and top with the sautéed apple filling.

Avocado Meyer Lemon Toast

Cooking time: 3 minutes

Preparation time: 10 minutes

Servings: 2

Nutrition facts: Calories 72, Total fat 2g, Protein 6g, Carbs 18g

Ingredients:

- 1/2 avocado
- 1/4 teaspoon of Meyer lemon zest
- 1 pinch of fine sea salt
- 2 slices of whole-grain bread
- 1/4 teaspoon of chia seeds
- 2 tablespoons of fresh cilantro chopped
- 1 pinch of cayenne pepper
- 1 teaspoon of Meyer lemon juice

Instructions:

Follow the instructions below to make avocado Meyer lemon toast.

1. Toast the slices of bread for around 3 to 4 minutes
2. In a medium-sized mixing dish, mash the avocado & add the cilantro, Meyer lemon juice, cayenne pepper, Meyer lemon zest, and salt. Spread the avocado mixture on the toast and sprinkle the chia seeds on top.

Low-Carb Breakfast Spinach Smoothie

Cooking time: 5 minutes

Preparation time: 5 minutes

Servings: 2

Nutrition facts: Calories 236, Total fat 11g, Protein 11g, Carbs 11g

Ingredients:

- 1/2 cup of low-fat plain Greek yogurt
- 1 cups of fresh spinach
- 1 cup of ice
- 2 tablespoons of nut butter of choice
- 1/4 cup of almond milk
- 1 teaspoon of vanilla extract
- 1/2 pitted avocado

Instructions:

Follow the instructions below to make a low-carb breakfast spinach smoothie.

1. In a blender, combine all of the ingredients except for the ice.
2. Blend until completely smooth.
3. Add and pulse in the ice cubes until they are completely crushed. Blend until the smoothie becomes smooth and creamy.

Breakfast Mushroom Surprise

Cooking time: 15 minutes

Preparation time: 10 minutes

Servings: 2

Nutrition facts: Calories 184, Total fat 18g, Protein 5g, Carbs 4g

Ingredients:

- 4 teaspoons of olive oil
- 2 Portobello mushrooms
- 1 tablespoon of finely grated cheddar cheese
- Salt and pepper
- 1 teaspoon of finely chopped garlic
- 2 large-sized eggs
- 1 teaspoon of dried thyme or rosemary

Instructions:

Follow the instructions below to make a breakfast mushroom surprise.

1. At 390°F, preheat the oven.
2. Arrange the mushrooms on a foil-lined roasting pan. Add the garlic, salt, & pepper to the mushrooms.
3. Bake for around 10 minutes or until soft.
4. Meanwhile, beat the eggs in a bowl, then season to taste with salt and pepper.
5. Cook the egg in a frying pan with the olive oil on low to medium heat. Cook, stirring slowly until the egg is fully cooked and set.
6. Quarter of the egg mixture should be spooned over each mushroom once they've been cooked. Sprinkle with cheese and thyme/rosemary on top. Serve right away.

Breakfast Barley Porridge

Cooking time: 15 minutes

Preparation time: 10 minutes

Servings: 4

Nutrition facts: Calories 189, Total fat 3g, Protein 7g, Carbs 23g

Ingredients:

- 28 g of sultanas
- 475 ml of almond milk unsweetened
- 1 tablespoon of flaked almonds
- 80 g of barley flakes
- 1 tablespoon of pumpkin seeds
- 21 g of agave nectar
- 1 teaspoon of ground cinnamon
- 2 tablespoons of sunflower seeds
- 1teaspoon of vanilla essence or vanilla bean

Instructions:

Follow the instructions below to make a breakfast barley porridge.

1. Heat the milk, together with the sweetener, nutmeg, cinnamon, and vanilla bean/essence, in a saucepan.
2. In a small-sized saucepan, combine the barley flakes & sultanas and cook for around 10 minutes on low heat.
3. Stir the mixture until the barley softens and it thickens.
4. In a nonstick frying pan, toast the flaked almonds, sunflower seeds, & pumpkin seeds until lightly toasted.
5. Cook for another 2 minutes after adding the seeds and nuts to the milk, ensuring everything is well blended.
6. Allow it cool for 2 minutes after removing from the heat.

Cheddar Breakfast Muffins

Cooking time: 15 minutes

Preparation time: 10 minutes

Servings: 4

Nutrition facts: Calories 510, Total fat 36g, Protein 20g, Carbs 30.6g

Ingredients:

- 2 large eggs free range
- 3 teaspoons of baking power
- 100 g of self-rising flour
- 1/2 teaspoon of salt
- 100 g of almond flour
- 50 g of butter
- 200 g of finely grated vegetarian cheddar cheese
- Pinch of ground pepper
- 200 ml of milk semi-skimmed

Instructions:

Follow the instructions below to make cheddar breakfast muffins.

1. At 400°F, preheat the oven and line a baking sheet with 12 muffin tins.
2. In a mixing dish, sift together the self-rising flour & baking powder, then add the cheese, almond flour, salt, & pepper.
3. In a saucepan, melt the butter and set it aside to cool few minutes.
4. In a separate dish, whisk together the milk and eggs, then gradually add the butter. Continue whisking until the entire mixture is the same in color.
5. Gradually pour the liquid mixture into the dry mixture, constantly whisking until the consistency is uniform. If the

mixture appears curdled, stir in a little bit of flour until it is smooth again.
6. Fill the muffin tins halfway with the batter and bake for 12 minutes.

English Breakfast Scones

Cooking time: 20 minutes

Preparation time: 10 minutes

Servings: 12

Nutrition facts: Calories 249, Total fat 15g, Protein 2g, Carbs 27g

Ingredients:

- 100 g of butter
- 1 teaspoon of vanilla essence
- 2 teaspoons of bicarb of soda
- 1 tablespoon of honey
- 200 g of almond flour
- 100 ml of apple juice unsweetened
- 2 tablespoons of Stevia
- 4 tablespoons of almond milk unsweetened
- 200 g of self-rising flour
- 100 g of raisins

Instructions:

Follow the instructions below to make English breakfast scones.

1. At 390°F, preheat the oven.
2. Honey, almond milk, unsweetened apple juice, butter, and vanilla essence should all be mixed together.
3. To make the dough, combine the self-rising flour, raisins, almond flour, bicarbonate of soda, and Stevia.
4. Roll out the dough to about an inch and a half thick on a lightly floured board. Using a pastry cutter, cut out circular shapes and set them on a greased baking tray.
5. Roll any remaining dough scraps together and continue until the entire mixture has been used. Bake for approximately 20 minutes.

6. Poke a skewer or something similarly long and thin into one of the scones to see whether it's done, then remove it.

Tasty Breakfast Egg Wraps

Cooking time: 8 minutes

Preparation time: 5 minutes

Servings: 4

Nutrition facts: Calories 429, Total fat 20g, Protein 28g, Carbs 31g

Ingredients:

- 10 medium-sized eggs
- 500 g of mushrooms pack closed cup
- 2 finely chopped generous handfuls of parsley
- 4 teaspoons of rapeseed oil + 2 drops
- 4 teaspoons of English mustard powder made using the water
- 320 g of halved cherry tomatoes
- 8 tablespoons of porridge oats

Instructions:

Follow the instructions below to make tasty breakfast egg wraps.

1. Half of the carton of mushrooms should be thickly sliced. In a nonstick pan, heat 2 teaspoons of rapeseed oil. Add the mushrooms, stir slightly, and cook for 6-8 minutes with the lid on the pan. Cook for another 1-2 minutes with the lid off until the tomatoes have softened.
2. Combine the eggs, parsley, and oats in a large-sized mixing bowl. In a big nonstick frying pan, heat a drop of oil. Pour in a quarter of the egg mixture and fry for 1 minute, or until almost set, then flip like a pancake. Remove from the pan, smear with a quarter of the mustard, then spoon a quarter of the filling down the center before rolling it up. Make a second wrap with the remaining egg mixture and stuffing.

Quinoa Berry Breakfast

Cooking time: 20 minutes

Preparation time: 5 minutes

Servings: 4

Nutrition facts: Calories 222, Total fat 4g, Protein 2g, Carbs 36g

Ingredients:

- 200 ml of water
- 100 g of blueberries
- 150 g of quinoa
- 100 g of strawberries
- 600 ml unsweetened almond milk
- 2 tablespoons of desiccated coconut

Instructions:

Follow the instructions below to make a quinoa berry breakfast. Roughly chop the nuts.

1. In a saucepan, bring the quinoa, milk, and water to a boil. Then reduce to medium heat & continue to cook for around 15 minutes.
2. Mix in the desiccated coconut thoroughly.
3. Divide the mixture among four bowls and top with blueberries and strawberries to serve.

Pepper Fajitas and Marinated Steak

Cooking time: 20 minutes

Preparation time: 10 minutes

Servings: 8

Per serving: Calories 375, Total fat 14g, Protein 29g, Carbs 29g

Ingredients:

- 4 sliced garlic cloves
- 3/4 teaspoon of pepper
- 1/2 cup of reduced-sodium beef or chicken broth
- 1 sweet onion large, make
- 3/4-inch-thick slices
- 8 warmed whole wheat tortillas 8 inches
- 1teaspoon of grated lime zest
- 4 halved and seeded jalapeno peppers
- 1/2 cup of fresh lime juice
- 1/2 cup of grated Mexican cheese blend
- 1 teaspoon of chili powder
- 1-1/2 pounds of flank steak or beef skirt steaks
- 3/4 teaspoon of salt
- 4 halved and seeded poblano or sweet red peppers

Instructions:

Follow the instructions below to make pepper fajitas and marinated steak.

1. Combine the 1/2 cup of broth, grated lime zest, fresh lime juice, garlic cloves, chili powder, pepper, and salt mixing bowl. Divide the mixture into two large-sized bowls. In a separate bowl, combine the peppers and onion and toss lightly to coat. Half the skirt steaks and place them in the second bowl; turn to coat. Refrigerate the vegetables and beef for at least 8 hours or overnight.

2. Remove the vegetables and beef from the marinade and discard them. Cover and grill the onion and poblanos on medium heat until tender, about 4-6 minutes per side. Jalapenos should be grilled until crisp-tender, about 2-3 minutes per side. Grill steaks, covered, on medium heat for 4-6 minutes per side, or until the desired doneness is reached. Allow 5 minutes for the steaks to rest.
3. Peppers should be thinly sliced, and onion should be coarsely chopped. Thinly slice steaks across the grain. Top tortillas with vegetables and beef, then cheese.

Diabetic Two Minutes Breakfast Smoothie

Cooking time: 0 minutes

Preparation time: 5 minutes

Servings: 2

Per serving: Calories 156, Total fat 3g, Protein 4g, Carbs 25g

Ingredients:

- 1 tablespoon of porridge oats
- 150 ml of skimmed milk
- 1 teaspoon of vanilla extract
- 1 frozen banana chunks
- 80 g of soft fruits whatever is available-blueberries, strawberries and mango will work well
- 5 to 6 drops of liquid stevia

Instructions:

Follow the instructions below to make diabetic two minutes' breakfast smoothie.

1. In a blender, combine all of the ingredients and blend for 1 minute, or until smooth. To serve, divide the banana oat smoothie between two glasses.

Delicious Breakfast Burrito

Cooking time: 10 minutes

Preparation time: 5 minutes

Servings: 1

Per serving: Calories 366, Total fat 21g, Protein 16g, Carbs 26g

Ingredients:

- 1 teaspoon of rapeseed oil
- 7 halved cherry tomatoes
- 1 teaspoon of chipotle paste
- 1 warmed whole-meal tortilla wrap
- 1 egg
- 50 g of kale
- 1/2 small sliced avocado

Instructions:

Follow the instructions below to make a delicious breakfast burrito.

1. In a jug, combine the chipotle paste, egg, & seasonings. In a large-sized frying pan, heat the oil and add the tomatoes and kale.
2. Push everything to the side of the pan once the kale has wilted and the tomatoes have softened. Scramble the beaten egg in the half of the pan that has been cleared. Fill the center of the wrap with everything, layer the top with avocado, wrap it up, and enjoy it right away.

Oat, Almond, And Raspberry Breakfast Cookies

Cooking time: 15 minutes

Preparation time: 10 minutes

Servings: 12 cookies

Per serving: Calories 86, Total fat 3g, Protein 2g, Carbs 13g

Ingredients:

- 150 g of porridge oats
- 1/2 teaspoon of cinnamon
- 2 mashed ripe bananas
- 100 g of frozen fresh raspberries
- 2 tablespoons of ground almonds

Instructions:

Follow the instructions below to make oat, almond, and raspberry breakfast cookies.

1. At 400°F, preheat the oven and line two baking pans with parchment paper. To produce a sticky dough, combine the banana, cinnamon, oats, almonds, and a bit of salt in a mixing bowl. Gently fold in the raspberries, being careful not to split them up. Scoop tablespoons of the mixture and roll them into balls, then lay them on a baking tray and flatten them with your hand.
2. Bake for 15 minutes, or until the cookies are golden brown and hard around the edges. Allow cooling. Keeps for up to three days in an airtight container.

Low-Carb Healthy Breakfast Smoothie

Cooking time: 0 minutes

Preparation time: 5 minutes

Servings: 2

Per serving: Calories 560, Total fat 48g, Protein 15g, Carbs 27g

Ingredients:

- 2 scoops of protein powder
- 1 cup of almond milk
- 1/4 teaspoon of vanilla extract
- 5 to 6 drops of liquid stevia, optional
- 3/4 cup of frozen mixed berries
- 1/2 cup of desiccated coconut
- 1/4 cup of water
- 1 tablespoon of flaxseed oil
- 1/4 teaspoon of ground cinnamon

Instructions:

Follow the instructions below to make a low-carb, healthy breakfast smoothie. Blend everything together in a blender until smooth.

1. You're ready to go once you've poured the mixture into a glass.

Breakfast Apple Muffins Diabetic-Friendly

Cooking time: 20 minutes

Preparation time: 10 minutes

Servings: 12

Per serving: Calories 98, Total fat 5g, Protein 8g, Carbs 16g

Ingredients:

- 2/3 cup of skim milk
- Vegetable oil cooking spray
- 21/2 teaspoons of baking powder
- 1 teaspoon of ground cinnamon
- 1 lightly beaten egg
- 1 cup of apple minced
- 1 2/3 cups of all-purpose flour
- 1/4 cup of melted margarine reduced-calorie
- 1/2 teaspoon of sea salt
- 1 tablespoon of stevia sugar substitute
- 1/4 teaspoon of nutmeg

Instructions:

Follow the instructions below to make breakfast apple muffins diabetic-friendly. At 400°F, preheat the oven. Spray 12 muffin tins with nonstick cooking spray.

1. In a large-sized mixing bowl, combine flour, baking powder, sea salt, stevia, cinnamon, and nutmeg. In a separate bowl, whisk together the skim milk, egg, & melted margarine; add to the flour mixture and stir just until the dry ingredients are moistened. Gently mix the apple mince into the batter. Fill muffin cups halfway with batter.
2. Bake for about 20 minutes in a preheated oven until the tops are gently browned.

Coconut Banana and Blueberry Porridge

Cooking time: 20 minutes

Preparation time: 5 minutes

Servings: 4

Per serving: Calories 227, Total fat 5g, Protein 6g, Carbs 38g

Ingredients:

- 150 ml of water
- 1 teaspoon of ground cinnamon
- 1 sliced banana, medium
- 100 g of quinoa
- 25 g of dried cranberries
- 350 g of almond milk unsweetened
- 1 tablespoon of coconut shavings
- 100 g of blueberries
- 50g of unsalted pistachio kernels

Instructions:

Follow the instructions below to make coconut banana and blueberry porridge.

1. In a saucepan, bring the quinoa, milk & water to a boil. Then reduce to medium heat & continue to cook for 15 minutes.
2. Add the blueberries and cranberries to the mix. Mix in the ground cinnamon until everything is well combined.
3. Pistachio kernels, coconut shavings, and banana slices should be scattered over the mixture in 4 breakfast bowls.

Breakfast Omega Seed Starter

Cooking time: 20 minutes

Preparation time: 5 minutes

Servings: 4

Per serving: Calories 160, Total fat 6g, Protein 5g, Carbs 23g

Ingredients:

- 100 ml of water
- 1/2 tablespoon of coconut oil
- 1/2 teaspoon of vanilla essence
- 2 tablespoons of omega seeds
- 100 g of quinoa
- 300 ml of fresh almond milk
- 1/4 teaspoon of cinnamon
- Splash of fresh lemon juice
- 1 tablespoon of honey

Instructions:

Follow the instructions below to make a breakfast omega seed starter.

1. Combine the water, milk, and quinoa in a medium-sized saucepan.
2. Then, bring the pan to a boil and reduce to low heat for 15 minutes.
3. Mix in the vanilla extract, coconut oil, lemon juice, & honey, then spoon into breakfast bowls. Toss in some omega seeds and enjoy!

Fruity Nutty Breakfast Yogurt

Cooking time: 0 minutes

Preparation time: 30 minutes

Servings: 4

Per serving: Calories 261, Total fat 11g, Protein 11g, Carbs 33g

Ingredients:

- 25 g of sultanas
- 400 g of soy yogurt unsweetened
- 4 dates
- 50 g of almonds & cashews
- 100 g of rolled oats

Instructions:

Follow the instructions below to make a fruity nutty breakfast yogurt.

1. In a large-sized mixing dish, combine the yogurt, two-thirds of the nuts, as well as the majority of the sultanas.
2. Set aside for 30 minutes in the refrigerator.
3. Remove the mixture from the fridge and whisk in the rolled oats well. Sprinkle with sultanas, almonds, and dates before serving!

Spinach with Poached Eggs

Cooking time: 10 minutes

Preparation time: 5 minutes

Servings: 1

Per serving: Calories 151, Total fat 10g, Protein 9g, Carbs 10g

Ingredients:

- 8 large eggs free-range
- Sea salt & black pepper, to taste
- 200 g of spinach
- 1/2 tablespoon of vegetable oil

Instructions:

Follow the instructions below to make spinach with poached eggs.

1. Fill a pot halfway with water and set it on medium heat until it starts to boil.
2. When the water has reached to boil, crack the egg and carefully pour it into the saucepan, making sure it is completely submerged.
3. Poaching the egg will take 1-2 minutes.
4. Cook the spinach in a frying pan with a little olive oil for 3 minutes while the eggs are poaching.
5. Serve the wilted spinach with an egg on top on a serving platter.

Kale and Pineapple Breakfast Smoothie

Cooking time: 0 minutes

Preparation time: 5 minutes

Servings: 2

Per serving: Calories 206, Total fat 7g, Protein 18g, Carbs 36g

Ingredients:

- 1 1/2 cups of pineapple cubed
- 1 cucumber
- 1cup of 0% fat Greek yogurt
- 3 cups of baby kale
- 2 tablespoons of hemp seeds

Instructions:

Follow the instructions below to make a kale and pineapple breakfast smoothie.

1. In a blender, combine all of the ingredients & blend until the smoothie is smooth and even.

Dip Recipes

Tasty Cranberry Sauce

Cooking time: 10 minutes

Preparation time: 5 minutes

Servings: 16

Per serving: Calories 3, Total fat 0g, Protein 0.1g, Carbs 8g

Ingredients:

- 2 teaspoons of minced ginger
- 400 g of fresh cranberries
- 2 teaspoons of ground cinnamon
- Zest & juice of a large orange
- 75 g of Stevia

Instructions:

Follow the instructions below to make a tasty cranberry sauce. In a food processor, puree the cranberries.

1. In a saucepan, place the cranberries.
2. Add the orange zest & juice, as well as the cinnamon and Stevia.
3. Bring the mixture to a boil and then reduce to a low flame for 7 minutes.
4. Your cranberry sauce is now ready to eat!

Mexican-Style Tomato Salsa

Cooking time: 0 minutes

Preparation time: 10 minutes

Servings: 4

Per serving: Calories 24, Total fat 0g, Protein 8g, Carbs 5g

Ingredients:

- 1 finely chopped red onion
- 1 teaspoon of finely chopped coriander
- 1 finely chopped red chili
- 4 ripe vine tomatoes Salt to taste
- 1teaspoon of finely chopped garlic
- 1/2 lime juice

Instructions:

Follow the instructions below to make a Mexican-style tomato salsa. Chop the tomatoes finely.

1. Mix in the remaining ingredients thoroughly.
2. To make a finer salsa, combine all of the ingredients in the food processor & pulse until smooth.
3. Serve with grilled or barbecued meats and veggies.

Peanut Satay Dip

Cooking time: 10 minutes

Preparation time: 5 minutes

Servings: 4

Per serving: Calories 73, Total fat 9g, Protein 6g, Carbs 1g

Ingredients:

- 2 finely chopped cloves of garlic
- 1 tablespoon of light soy sauce
- 6 finely chopped shallots
- 1 finely chopped red chili
- 2 tablespoons of dark soy sauce
- 1 teaspoon of finely chopped coriander
- 1 teaspoon of finely chopped ginger
- 1teaspoon of sesame oil
- 2 tablespoons of crunchy peanut butter
- 1 lime juice

Instructions:

Follow the instructions below to make a peanut satay dip. On medium heat, heat the oil.

1. Sauté the shallots until they are golden brown in color.
2. Reduce the flame to low and add the ginger, garlic, chili powder, peanut butter, soy sauces, and sesame oil.
3. Cook for a few minutes or until the mixture is completely smooth. If the mixture becomes too thick, thin it up with a little water.
4. Add the coriander and lime juice when the mixture has cooled.

Harissa and Black-Eyed Bean Dip

Cooking time: 0 minutes

Preparation time: 10 minutes

Servings: 4

Per serving: Calories 147, Total fat 1g, Protein 7g, Carbs 20.1g

Ingredients:

- 2 cloves of finely chopped garlic
- 1/2 teaspoon of Harissa paste
- 1 1/2 tablespoons of extra virgin olive oil
- 400 g of black-eyed beans, drained & rinsed
- 50 g of flat-leaf parsley
- 1 red onion small
- Juice of 1 lemon

Instructions:

Follow the instructions below to make harissa and black-eyed bean dip.

1. In a food processor, combine the black-eyed beans, parsley, garlic, onion, and Harissa paste. Whizz in the lemon juice and olive oil until smooth.
2. It's done when the mixture is gritty.
3. Cucumber, raw cauliflower, & raw broccoli pair beautifully with this dip.

Tasty Homemade Hummus Dip

Cooking time: 0 minutes

Preparation time: 10 minutes

Servings: 4

Per serving: Calories 180.3, Total fat 16g, Protein 8g, Carbs 12g

Ingredients:

- 3 tablespoons of tahini
- 2 tablespoons of fresh lemon juice
- 250 g of tinned chickpeas, drained & rinsed
- Salt to taste
- 2 crushed cloves garlic
- 3 tablespoons of sesame oil
- 1 teaspoon of paprika

Instructions:

Follow the instructions below to make a tasty homemade hummus dip.

1. In a blender or food processor, combine all of the ingredients.
2. If the mix is too dry, add a little additional oil or water. Serve with crudités of vegetables.

Simple Pea Dip

Cooking time: 10 minutes

Preparation time: 5 minutes

Servings: 4

Per serving: Calories 232, Total fat 17g, Protein 5g, Carbs 15g

Ingredients:

- 2 tablespoons of almond butter
- 1 lemon juice
- 50 g of feta cheese
- 300 g of frozen peas
- 2 finely chopped cloves of garlic
- 3 tablespoons of olive oil
- 5 sprigs of thyme

Instructions:

Follow the instructions below to make a simple pea dip. Boil peas until they are soft.

1. Then, combine the peas, almond butter, lemon juice, garlic, thyme, and olive oil in a blender. Blend till the mixture is completely smooth.
2. Serve with a choice of crudités, such as carrots & celery, and crumbled feta cheese on top.

Simple Mint Yogurt Dip

Cooking time: 0 minutes

Preparation time: 5 minutes

Servings: 4

Per serving: Calories 43, Total fat 0.9g, Protein 5g, Carbs 4g

Ingredients:

- 1 tablespoon of mint sauce
- 200 ml of plain yogurt low-fat

Instructions:

Follow the instructions below to make a simple mint yogurt dip.

1. In a mixing dish, combine the yogurt and the mint sauce.
2. Now, the dip is ready to eat.

Greek-Style Aubergine Dip

Cooking time: 20 minutes

Preparation time: 10 minutes

Servings: 1

Per serving: Calories 32, Total fat 1g, Protein 1g, Carbs 2g

Ingredients:

- 2 garlic bulbs large
- 120 ml of red capsicum very finely diced
- 2 tablespoons of olive oil
- 680 g of aubergines
- 1teaspoon of sea salt unrefined
- 2 tablespoons of fresh lemon juice

Instructions:

Follow the instructions below to make Greek-style aubergine dip.

1. At 475°F, preheat the oven.
2. In a glass baking dish, place the whole aubergines & garlic bulbs.
3. Place the baking dish in the oven for 20 minutes or until the vegetables are totally soft. Remove the pans from the oven & set them aside to cool completely.
4. Remove the soft flesh from the aubergines and put it in a large mixing dish. Remove the peels & throw them away.
5. Remove the garlic bulbs' outer peels and toss them out. Squeeze the soft meat off the garlic cloves and place it in the large mixing dish where the aubergine flesh was placed.
6. Combine the olive oil, salt, and lemon juice.
7. In a blender, puree the ingredients until it's perfectly smooth and velvety. Mix in the diced capsicum with a spoon until thoroughly combined.

8. 1Allow to sit in the fridge for a few hours, well covered, to develop the flavors.

Delicious Ranch Dip

Cooking time: 0 minutes

Preparation time: 5 minutes

Servings: 4

Per serving: Calories 128, Total fat 4g, Protein 5g, Carbs 18g

Ingredients:

- 2 teaspoons of garlic powder
- 1 teaspoon of ground pepper
- 2 tablespoons of dried parsley
- 1 teaspoon of sea salt
- 5 teaspoons of dried dill
- 1 cup of Greek yogurt
- 2 teaspoons of onion powder
- 1 teaspoon of dried chives

Veggies:

- 1 sliced carrot
- 1sliced Lebanese/ English cucumber
- 2 thin slices of sticks celery

Instructions:

Follow the instructions below to make a delicious ranch dip.

1. Combine all seasonings in a sealed jar and store.
2. Use 1 to 2 teaspoons of seasoning per cup of yogurt.
3. Combine all ingredients in a mixing bowl & serve with chopped vegetables of your choice!

Tasty Dill Dip

Cooking time: 0 minutes

Preparation time: 15 minutes

Servings: 21

Per serving: Calories 55, Total fat 4g, Protein 1g, Carbs 2g

Ingredients:

- 2 teaspoons of parsley flakes
- 1 1/3 cups of sour cream fat-free
- 1 teaspoon of garlic powder
- 3 drops of hot sauce
- 1 1/3 cups of mayonnaise reduced-fat
- 1 teaspoon of dill weed
- 1 teaspoon of seasoned salt
- 2 teaspoons of dry onions

Instructions:

Follow the instructions below to make a tasty dill dip.

1. In a mixing dish, combine sour cream & mayonnaise.
2. Mix in the remaining ingredients thoroughly.
3. Refrigerate the dip for at least 2 hours to allow flavors to combine. Serve with a variety of crisp veggies on the side.

Vegetarian Recipes

Tasty Veggie Shepherd's Pie

Cooking time: 25 minutes

Preparation time: 5 minutes

Servings: 4

Per serving: Calories 294, Total fat 8g, Protein 28g, Carbs 23g

Ingredients:

- 5 washed, peeled & chopped medium carrots
- 1 tablespoon of tomato puree
- 250 g of vegetarian mince
- 1 finely chopped onion
- Salt & freshly ground pepper for taste
- 1 washed, peeled & cubed medium potato
- 20 roughly chopped button mushrooms
- 1 tablespoon of vegetable oil
- 200 g of finely chopped tomatoes
- 75 g of finely grated cheddar cheese

Instructions:

Follow the instructions below to make a tasty veggie shepherd's pie.

1. At 400°F, preheat the oven.
2. Boil together the potato & carrots for about 5 minutes, or until they are soft. Sauté the onions in the oil till they are golden brown, about 5 minutes.
3. Cook for a few minutes after adding the vegetable mince.
4. Cook for yet another 3 minutes after adding the mushrooms, tomatoes, and tomato puree. Season with salt and pepper to taste.
5. Place the whole thing in an oven-safe dish.
6. In a colander, combine the potatoes and carrots. Then add the cheese and mash it all together.

7. Season with salt and pepper and serve over the mince mixture. 1Bake in the oven for about 20 minutes, or until done.
8. 1Remove the dish from the oven when it is hot. Allow cooling slightly before serving!

Simple Grilled Aubergine

Cooking time: 10 minutes

Preparation time: 5 minutes

Servings: 4

Per serving: Calories 194, Total fat 18g, Protein 8g, Carbs 16g

Ingredients:

- 250 g of natural yogurt low-fat
- 1 lemon juice
- 2 large sliced aubergines
- Salt & pepper to season
- 2 tablespoons of olive oil
- 3tablespoons of tahini paste
- 1 tablespoon of mixed herbs coriander, parsley & mint
- 3 finely chopped garlic cloves

Instructions:

Follow the instructions below to make a simple grilled aubergine.

1. Season each aubergine slice with a drizzle of olive oil.
2. Preheat the grill or griddle pan.
3. Grill the aubergine slices from both sides for a minute or two once the barbeque or pan is hot. Season the yogurt with the tahini paste, lemon juice, garlic, and herbs.

Halloumi and Quinoa Salad

Cooking time: 10 minutes

Preparation time: 5 minutes

Servings: 2

Per serving: Calories 585, Total fat 42g, Protein 22g, Carbs 20.3g

Ingredients:

- 3 tablespoons of olive oil
- 5 g of ground cumin
- 6 sun-dried tomatoes
- 85 g of quinoa
- 1thinly sliced small red onion
- 200 g of sliced halloumi
- 2 teaspoons of red wine vinegar

Instructions:

Follow the instructions below to make a halloumi and quinoa salad.

1. Cook the quinoa per the package directions, drain well, and add in a mixing dish.
2. Mix the cumin, red onion, sun-dried tomatoes, red wine vinegar, and olive oil.
3. In a griddle pan, cook the halloumi until it becomes soft, about 3 to 4 minutes.
4. Put the halloumi over the quinoa on a platter and serve right away.

Leek and Sun Roasted Tomatoes Frittata

Cooking time: 15 minutes

Preparation time: 5 minutes

Servings: 2

Per serving: Calories 311, Total fat 53g, Protein 16g, Carbs 23g

Ingredients:

- 6 sliced sun roasted tomatoes
- 1 sliced leek
- Salt & freshly ground black pepper
- 1 tablespoon of olive oil
- 30 g of spinach frozen or fresh
- 4 eggs

Instructions:

Follow the instructions below to make leek and sun roasted tomatoes frittata.

1. Cook until the leeks are soft in a medium-sized nonstick frying pan with olive oil.
2. Then add the spinach & tomatoes salt and pepper to taste and cook till the spinach is wilted. Whisk the eggs separately & pour them into the pan, coating most of the other ingredients.
3. Gently move around the sides of the pan as the eggs cook to enable the uncooked egg on top to cook in the bottom of the pan.
4. Once the frittata is done through, place it on the grill to crisp up at the top without scorching the bottom.
5. Enjoy by slicing it into slices.

Carrot and Chickpea Stew

Cooking time: 25 minutes

Preparation time: 5 minutes

Servings: 2

Per serving: Calories 356, Total fat 7g, Protein 51g, Carbs 16g

Ingredients:
- 100 g of spinach
- 2 chopped celery sticks
- 1 tablespoon of olive oil
- 1/2 teaspoon of ground ginger
- 1 sliced red onion
- 140 g of chopped carrots
- 1 teaspoon of ground coriander
- 1 tablespoon of tomato purée
- Ground paprika
- 1 teaspoon of ground cumin
- 2 chopped cloves of garlic
- 400 g of chickpeas
- 1 tablespoon of crème fraiche
- 400 g of chopped tomatoes
- 1/2 teaspoon of turmeric
- 1 bay leaf
- 1/2 teaspoon of cayenne pepper

Instructions:

Follow the instructions below to make a carrot and chickpea stew.

1. In a frying pan, warm the olive oil and add the garlic, onions, and celery. Cook for around 5 minutes
2. Add the remaining of ingredients excluding the crème fraiche & paprika.

3. Check that the carrots are cooked after 20 minutes of infusing on low to medium heat. With the dollop of crème fraiche and a sprinkling of paprika, serve.

Miso and Mushroom Broth

Cooking time: 25 minutes

Preparation time: 5 minutes

Servings: 2

Per serving: Calories 492, Total fat 42g, Protein 95g, Carbs 29g

Ingredients:

- 75 g of rice noodles
- 50 g of broken up enoki mushrooms
- 1 tablespoon of olive oil
- 3 teaspoons of soy sauce
- 1tablespoon of miso paste
- 125 g of Shiitake mushrooms
- 50 g of finely sliced mange tout
- Chopped fresh coriander
- 2 finely sliced shallots
- 300 ml of hot chicken stock
- 25 g of button mushrooms
- 2 teaspoons of rice vinegar
- 100 g of baby spinach

Instructions:

Follow the instructions below to make a miso and mushroom broth.

1. In a nonstick wok, add the oil and heat it.
2. Add the shallots to the wok & cook for 5 minutes, or until tender. Combine the mange tout, mushrooms, & spinach.
3. Cook for another 5 minutes in a stir-fry pan.
4. Add the rice vinegar, soy sauce, and miso paste to the heated stock in the pan. To mix the flavors, whisk together all of the ingredients.
5. Allow for a 10-minute simmer to ensure that everything is done through. Finally, add the noodles & coriander to the

wok and cook for a few minutes more. In large soup bowls, serve.

Winter Chili Vegetable

Cooking time: 25 minutes

Preparation time: 5 minutes

Servings: 2

Per serving: Calories 489, Total fat 30.8g, Protein 9g, Carbs 29g

Ingredients:

- 2 tablespoons of olive oil
- 70 g of chopped carrots
- 80 g of diced swede
- 400 g of chopped tomatoes
- 1 teaspoon of ground cumin
- 75 g of diced celeriac
- 400 g of mixed beans or kidney beans
- 1 tablespoon of tomato purée
- 2 crushed cloves of garlic
- 1 bay leaf
- 1sliced leek
- 60 g of chopped celery
- 1 sliced red onion

Instructions:

Follow the instructions below to make a winter chili vegetable.

1. To soften the celeriac, carrots, and swede, boil them in salty water for 5 minutes.
2. Add the onion, leek, garlic, and celery to a frying pan on medium heat and cook for 4 minutes. In a saucepan, combine the parboiled veggies & onion mixture.
3. Toss in the tomato can, bay leaf, tomato purée, and cumin. Allow for 15 minutes of simmering time.
4. Add the tin of drained & washed beans to the casserole dish and continue to cook for another 5 minutes.

5. Serve right away in hot bowls.

Delicious Okra Curry

Cooking time: 20 minutes

Preparation time: 5 minutes

Servings: 4

Per serving: Calories 320, Total fat 12g, Protein 8g, Carbs 43g

Ingredients:

- 2 teaspoons of finely chopped ginger
- 500 g of okra, cut into
- 1/2 inch slices
- 1 teaspoon of cumin seeds
- 100 g of finely chopped canned tomatoes
- 2 tablespoons of oil
- 8 whole wheat chapattis, ready to eat
- 1/2 teaspoon of mustard seeds
- Salt to taste
- 1/2 teaspoon of turmeric powder
- 4 finely chopped garlic cloves
- 1 finely chopped medium onion

Instructions:

Follow the instructions below to make a delicious okra curry.

1. Chop the okra into small pieces, about the size of a finger.
2. In a frying pan, add one tablespoon of oil and heat it on medium heat. Put the mustard seeds after the oil is heated.
3. Sprinkle the cumin seeds & turmeric powder once the seeds have popped. Remove after 30 seconds of cooking.
4. In a frying pan, heat the remaining tablespoon of oil. Fry for 4 minutes with the chopped onions, add garlic and ginger and cook for another minute.
5. In a food processor, blitz the tinned tomatoes.

6. In a large-sized saucepan, combine the mustard seed mixture, okra, and onion combination.
7. Toss in the tomatoes and season with salt to taste. The meal is ready to eat with whole wheat chapattis after 5 minutes of cooking!

Stir Fry Tangy Quorn

Cooking time: 10 minutes

Preparation time: 5 minutes

Servings: 4

Per serving: Calories 200, Total fat 6g, Protein 12g, Carbs 17g

Ingredients:

- 2 tablespoons of olive oil
- 400 g of Quorn pieces
- 1 finely chopped green chili
- 1 tablespoon of tomato sauce
- Salt to taste
- 1/2 tablespoon of soy sauce/coconut aminos
- 1 tablespoon of tandoori masala powder
- 1 tablespoon of agave nectar

Instructions:

Follow the instructions below to make a stir fry tangy Quorn.

1. For an hour, marinate the Quorn in tomato sauce, tandoori masala powder, soy sauce/coconut aminos, agave nectar, chili powder, and salt.
2. In a wok, warm the oil and stir-fried the Quorn until it is done around 8 to 10 minutes. Serve with boiling vegetables or your favorite salad!

Sweet & Sour Tofu

Cooking time: 10 minutes

Preparation time: 5 minutes

Servings: 2

Per serving: Calories 463, Total fat 19g, Protein 30.2g, Carbs 35g

Ingredients:

- 2 minced garlic cloves
- 1 red pepper, slice into 16 squares
- 400 g of tinned pineapple pieces, with
- 200 ml of juice set aside
- 1 tablespoon of sesame oil
- 2 teaspoons of minced ginger
- 1 tablespoon of soy sauce
- 450 g of drained & diced extra-firm tofu

Instructions:

Follow the instructions below to make sweet & sour tofu.

1. In a wok on medium heat, heat the sesame oil.
2. Cook for 2 minutes with the ginger and garlic.
3. Toss the tofu, pineapple pieces, red pepper, and soy sauce together. Cook for 3 to 5 minutes in a stir-fry pan.
4. Now it's time to serve the food!

Delicious Chickpea Curry

Cooking time: 20 minutes

Preparation time: 5 minutes

Servings: 4

Per serving: Calories 320, Total fat 9g, Protein 13g, Carbs 46g

Ingredients:
- 6 finely chopped garlic cloves
- 2 teaspoons of ground coriander
- 1 teaspoon of green chili
- 240 g of drained and rinsed tinned chickpeas
- 250 ml of water
- 1/2 teaspoon of turmeric powder
- 4 whole wheat chapattis ready to eat
- 1 finely chopped medium onion
- Salt to taste
- 1 teaspoon of garam masala
- 2 teaspoons of finely chopped ginger
- 2 teaspoons of amchoor powder
- 200 g of finely chopped canned tomatoes
- 1 tablespoon of vegetable oil

Instructions:

Follow the instructions below to make a delicious chickpea curry.

1. In a medium-sized frying pan, pour the oil & heat it on medium heat. Place the onions in the pan and cook for 4 minutes, or until golden brown. Cook for another 2 minutes after adding the ginger and garlic.
2. Combine the tomatoes, chili, amchoor powder, turmeric, ground coriander, and salt in a large- sized mixing dish. Cook for around 4 minutes.
3. Bring the water to a boil, then add the washed and drained chickpeas. Toss both ingredients into the frying pan.

4. Cover and stir. Eat with whole wheat chapattis after ten minutes of cooking.

Tasty Vegetable mince

Cooking time: 25 minutes

Preparation time: 5 minutes

Servings: 4

Per serving: Calories 370, Total fat 4g, Protein 21g, Carbs 55g

Ingredients:

- 2 chopped onions
- 1 tablespoon of tomato puree
- 400 g of veggie mince
- 1 tablespoon of olive oil
- 800 g of brown long grain rice cooked
- 100 g of per serving
- 400 g of finely chopped canned tomatoes
- 4 finely chopped cloves of garlic
- Season with salt & pepper
- 100ml of water

Instructions:

Follow the instructions below to make a tasty vegetable mince.

1. Four minutes on medium heat, sauté the onions & garlic in the olive oil.
2. Put veggie mince and cook for 4 to 5 minutes, or until the vegetarian mince is browned. Cook for 3 minutes after adding the tomatoes & tomato puree.
3. Add the water, cover the pan, and cook for about 10 minutes at low heat until the sauce is rich and creamy.
4. Season with salt and pepper to taste. Serve with brown rice.

Tempting Mutter Paneer

Cooking time: 25 minutes

Preparation time: 5 minutes

Servings: 4

Per serving: Calories 515, Total fat 26g, Protein 21g, Carbs 53g

Ingredients:

- 100 g of frozen peas
- 227 g of cubed paneer cheese
- 2 teaspoons of garam masala
- 1 teaspoon of finely chopped coriander
- 1 teaspoon of finely chopped ginger
- 1 tablespoon of olive oil for shallow frying paneer
- Salt to taste
- 1 finely chopped medium onion
- 1 teaspoon of cumin
- 400 g of finely chopped canned tomatoes
- 4 finely chopped garlic cloves
- 800 g of cooked brown rice for serving
- 1 finely chopped green chili
- 1 teaspoon of turmeric
- 1 tablespoon of olive oil for frying onions
- 250 ml of boiling water

Instructions:

Follow the instructions below to make tempting mutter paneer.

1. Place a frying pan on medium heat with a tablespoon of oil in it.
2. Add the paneer to the heated oil and cook till golden brown.
3. It should take about 6 to 8 minutes to complete this task.

4. If you don't turn the paneer numerous times while cooking, it'll split due to the water content. Place the cheese on the kitchen roll once it has browned.
5. In a medium-sized frying pan, pour the remaining tablespoon of oil. Add the onions to the heated oil and cook for 4 minutes.
6. Fry for 2 minutes after stirring in the ginger, chili, garlic, cumin, salt, garam masala, and turmeric.
7. Add the tomatoes, reduce the flame to low, and cook for 5 minutes. Add the paneer & peas to the boiling water.
8. Allow for a 5-minute simmer.
9. 1Make sure the peas are fully cooked before serving.

Tasty Kidney Bean Curry

Cooking time: 20 minutes

Preparation time: 5 minutes

Servings: 4

Per serving: Calories 274, Total fat 8g, Protein 12g, Carbs 35g

Ingredients:

- 6 finely chopped garlic cloves
- 2 tablespoons of olive oil
- 400 g of tinned tomatoes
- 1 finely chopped onion
- 800 g of tinned kidney beans
- 4 teaspoons of minced ginger

Instructions:

Follow the instructions below to make a tasty kidney bean curry. In a frying pan, pour the oil and heat it on medium heat.

1. Fry the onions, ginger, and garlic for 4 minutes once the oil has heated up. Cook for yet another 2 minutes after adding the canned tomatoes.
2. Allow the kidney beans to simmer for 5 to 8 minutes, along with the liquid from the can. Season to taste then serves in a bowl with a coriander garnish.

Falafel Burgers with Pita Bread

Cooking time: 15 minutes

Preparation time: 5 minutes

Servings: 4

Per serving: Calories 240, Total fat 7g, Protein 4g, Carbs 28g

Ingredients:

- 1 finely chopped red onion
- 2 teaspoons of ground cumin
- 5 tablespoons of plain flour
- 4 pitta bread toasted
- 10 g of flat-leaf parsley
- 200 g of tub tomato salsa for serving
- Salt to taste
- 200 g of rinsed & drained tinned chickpeas
- 2 finely chopped garlic cloves
- 1 teaspoon of ground coriander
- 5 tablespoons of olive oil

Instructions:

Follow the instructions below to make falafel burgers with pita bread.

1. Ensure that the chickpeas are well-drained.
2. In a food processor, whizz the chickpeas, red onion, garlic, flour, parsley, ground cumin, ground coriander, and salt to taste until the mixture is smooth.
3. With your hands, form the mixture into four patties.
4. Place a nonstick frying pan on medium flame and pour in the olive oil.
5. When the oil is hot, cook the burgers for around 3 minutes on each side, or until golden brown. Serve with tomato salsa or a green salad on a toasted pita and enjoy!

Spaghetti Bolognese Low-Carb

Cooking time: 25 minutes

Preparation time: 5 minutes

Servings: 4

Per serving: Calories 482, Total fat 17g, Protein 17g, Carbs 21g

Ingredients:

- 2 minced garlic cloves
- 400 ml of vegetable stock
- 3 tablespoons of olive oil
- Salt & freshly ground pepper to taste
- 1 diced medium onion
- 100 g of grated carrot
- 3 tablespoons of olive oil
- 2 x 400 g tins of chopped tomatoes
- 300 g pack of Quorn mince
- 4 courgettes medium for the courgette pasta

Instructions:

Follow the instructions below to make a spaghetti Bolognese low-carb.

1. In a large saucepan on medium heat, add 3 tablespoons of olive oil. Cook, occasionally stirring, for 4 to 5 minutes, or until the onion is transparent. Cook for another 2 minutes after adding the minced garlic.
2. Cook for yet another minute after adding the grated carrot.
3. Add the tomatoes to the pan & stir well. Bring the stock to a low boil, then reduce to low flame. Reduce the flame to low and cook for about 15 minutes, or until the sauce is thick and rich. Add the veggie mince halfway through the cooking process. To taste, season with salt & freshly ground pepper.

4. Use a spiralizer, a julienne peeler, or cut the courgette into extremely thin slices and then thin spaghetti-like strips to make the courgette. It is suitable for both hot and cold consumption. 3 tablespoons olive oil, 3-4 minutes to fry the courgette
5. Place the courgette in the base of your plate & top with a generous tablespoon of Bolognese sauce.

Tasty Vegetable Curry

Cooking time: 20 minutes

Preparation time: 5 minutes

Servings: 2

Per serving: Calories 328, Total fat 17g, Protein 4g, Carbs 37g

Ingredients:

- 2 teaspoons of finely chopped garlic
- 200 ml of hot vegetable stock
- 50 g of courgettes
- 250 g of tinned chickpeas
- 2 tablespoons of vegetable oil
- 1 teaspoon of turmeric powder
- Salt & freshly ground pepper to taste
- 1 finely sliced medium onion
- 2 teaspoons of finely chopped ginger
- 50 g of sugar snaps
- 250 g of finely chopped tinned tomatoes
- 50g of broccoli

Instructions:

Follow the instructions below to make a tasty vegetable curry.

1. In a large-sized saucepan on high heat, heat the oil. Cook the onions in a skillet for 5 minutes or until golden brown. Fry for another minute after adding the garlic and ginger. After that, stir in the turmeric powder thoroughly.
2. Add in the canned tomatoes with boiling vegetable stock.
3. Bring to a boil, then reduce the flame to low and add the broccoli, sugar snaps, courgettes, and chickpeas.
4. To taste, flavor the curry with salt & freshly ground pepper. After 7 minutes of cooking, your food is ready to eat!

Courgette Cheesy Frittata

Cooking time: 15 minutes

Preparation time: 5 minutes

Servings: 4

Per serving: Calories 267, Total fat 21g, Protein 12g, Carbs 4g

Ingredients:

- 250 g of finely sliced courgettes
- 30 g of finely grated hard vegetarian cheese
- 50 g of butter
- Salt & freshly ground pepper to taste
- 1 finely sliced medium onion
- 8 lightly beaten medium eggs

Instructions:

Follow the instructions below to make courgette cheesy frittata.

1. In a large-sized nonstick frying pan, melt 25g butter. The onion should be fried for 2 minutes. Place the sliced courgette in the pan & cook for 4 minutes, or until soft.
2. Start the grill.
3. In the same frying pan, melt the remaining 25 grams of butter.
4. Season the eggs to taste with salt and black pepper before pouring them into the frying pan & cooking them for 3 minutes.
5. Sprinkle the grated cheese over the frittata and place it on the prepared grill for 2 minutes or until it is totally set.
6. Cut the quarters in half and enjoy!

Delicious Cornmeal Flan

Cooking time: 25 minutes

Preparation time: 5 minutes

Servings: 6

Per serving: Calories 563, Total fat 43g, Protein 24g, Carbs 39g

Ingredients:

- 200 g of cornmeal
- 2 tablespoons of garlic
- 220 ml of milk semi-skimmed
- 1 finely chopped medium white onion
- 2 sliced medium tomatoes
- 1 teaspoon of red chili flakes
- 220 g of grated cheddar cheese
- 150 g of finely chopped plum tinned tomatoes
- Freshly ground salt & pepper
- 300 g of almond flour

Instructions:

Follow the instructions below to make a delicious cornmeal flan. At 360°F, preheat the oven.

1. Butter a 9-inch flan pan and line it with baking parchment.
2. In a large-sized mixing dish, combine the garlic, salt, chili flakes, and pepper.
3. Add in the milk, 200g cheddar cheese, cornmeal, finely chopped onion, almond flour, and tinned tomatoes.
4. Bake for around 20 to 25 minutes after pouring the ingredients into the flan shell. Add the sliced tomatoes on top.
5. Using a skewer, check if the flan is cooked. If it comes out clean, the flan is done to be taken from the oven.

6. To serve, add the rest of the cheddar cheese on top, slice, dish, and enjoy!

Cashew Vegetable Stir Fry

Cooking time: 15 minutes

Preparation time: 5 minutes

Servings: 2

Per serving: Calories 420, Total fat 28g, Protein 12g, Carbs 39g

Ingredients:

- 4 finely chopped garlic cloves
- 2 chopped medium carrots
- 1 chopped leek
- 150 g finely sliced greens
- 2 tablespoons of olive oil
- 75 g of peas
- 3 teaspoons of minced ginger
- 1 tablespoon of light soy sauce
- Salt to taste
- 2 chopped celery stalks
- 50 g unsalted cashew nuts
- 150g of chopped broccoli florets
- 2 sliced medium tomatoes

Instructions:

Follow the instructions below to make a cashew vegetable stir fry.

1. In a wok on high flame, pour the oil and cook the chopped leek for around 3 minutes. Stir in the garlic, ginger, and soy sauce for another 2 minutes.
2. Cook for another 2 minutes after adding the celery, carrots, peas, broccoli, and tomatoes. Cook for another minute after adding the greens & cashew nuts.
3. Serve immediately while still hot.

Appetizer And Snacks Recipes

Cream Cheese and Smoked Salmon Vol au vents

Cooking time: 15 minutes

Preparation time: 10 minutes

Servings: 16

Per serving: Calories 93, Total fat 6g, Protein 7g, Carbs 8g

Ingredients:

- 180 g of softened cream cheese
- 1 tablespoon of finely chopped fresh dill
- 16 vol-au-vent cases, ready to cook
- Dill sprigs, for serving
- 80 g of smoked salmon, slice into strips
- Ground black pepper for season
- 1 1/2 tablespoons of lemon juice

Instructions:

Follow the instructions below to make cream cheese and smoked salmon vol au vents. At 400°F, preheat the oven.

1. From frozen, bake your vol-au-vents for 15 minutes.
2. In the meantime, combine the lemon juice, cream cheese, & black pepper.
3. Fill each case with a heaping teaspoon of the cream cheese mix and shredded smoked salmon. Serve with a dill sprig as a garnish.

Tofu and Vegetable Wontons

Cooking time: 10 minutes

Preparation time: 10 minutes

Servings: 16

Per serving: Calories 113, Total fat 7g, Protein 1g, Carbs 15g

Ingredients:

For the Filling:

- 100 g of mashed firm tofu
- 1 finely sliced Pak Choi leaf
- 1 teaspoon of sesame oil
- 1 lightly beaten egg
- 3 finely chopped water chestnuts
- 1/4 teaspoon of salt
- 16 wonton wrappers, or as required
- Pinch of pepper
- 5 cups of vegetable oil for deep-frying, as required
- Finely sliced small white onion
- 2 teaspoons of grated carrots
- 2 teaspoons of grated ginger

For the Egg wash:

- 1 teaspoon of water 1 egg

Instructions:

Follow the instructions below to make tofu and vegetable wontons.

1. Season the egg with salt and black pepper after lightly beating it.
2. In a mixing dish, combine the mashed tofu with veggies white onion, Pak Choi, water chestnuts, carrots, and ginger.
3. In a frying pan, add the sesame oil and warm it on low heat.

4. To stuff the wontons, arrange a wrapper in a diamond shape in front of you. Apply egg wash to all sides with your finger.
5. Fill the center with a spoonful of filling.
6. To make a triangle, bend the wonton in 1/2 from one corner to the other.
7. Then, to produce the wonton form, squeeze the larger two triangle points together. Deep-fry the dumpling wrappers for approximately 2 minutes, or until golden and crispy.

Witches' Broomsticks Snack

Cooking time: 0 minutes

Preparation time: 10 minutes

Servings: 4

Per serving: Calories 89, Total fat 5g, Protein 7g, Carbs 5g

Ingredients:

- 4 twigs
- 4 strings of cheese

Instructions:

Follow the instructions below to make witches' broomsticks Snack.

1. To make the broom, cut off the tips of the cheese strings & fray the edges.
2. To symbolize the broomstick, insert twigs into the middle of a cheese string.

Tasty Granola Bars

Cooking time: 20 minutes

Preparation time: 10 minutes

Servings: 12

Per serving: Calories 170, Total fat 12g, Protein 3g, Carbs 18g

Ingredients:

- 5 tablespoons of agave nectar
- 110 g of butter
- 100 g of flaked almonds
- 120 g of rolled oats
- 50 g of Stevia
- 75 g of raisins

Instructions:

Follow the instructions below to make tasty granola bars. At 320°F, preheat the oven.

1. Melt the butter in a large-sized saucepan on low flame. After that, add the Stevia & agave nectar.
2. In a large-sized mixing dish, add the raisins, rolled oats, and flaked almonds. Now drizzle in the buttery syrup, making sure the oats are evenly coated.
3. Bake for around 20 minutes after pouring the granola ingredients into an 8x8 inch baking pan. These energy-packed granola bars make a fantastic snack.

Feta Spinach Rolls

Cooking time: 20 minutes

Preparation time: 10 minutes

Servings: 16

Per serving: Calories 102, Total fat 7g, Protein 4g, Carbs 17g

Ingredients:

For the Dough:

- 100 ml of lukewarm whole milk
- 1 yeast packet
- 250 g of whole wheat flour
- 1 lightly beaten large egg
- 40 g of wheat gluten
- 100 ml of lukewarm water
- A pinch of salt

For the Filling:

- 1/2 teaspoon of marjoram
- 330 g of spinach
- A pinch of freshly ground pepper
- 125 g of feta cheese crumbled
- A pinch of salt

Instructions:

Follow the instructions below to make feta spinach rolls.

1. At 400°F, preheat the oven for around 10 minutes, then turn it off.
2. Combine the gluten, whole-wheat flour, & salt in a medium-sized mixing dish. Set the mixture aside.
3. In the bowl of your mixer, mix the milk and water.

4. The yeast should then be sprinkled on top and thoroughly mixed. Whisk the egg until it is entirely mixed.
5. Mix in the flour mixture until it is well mixed.
6. Grease your hands and roll the dough into a smooth ball before placing it in a lightly greased basin.
7. Cover the bowl with foil and leave in the warm oven for 20 minutes, or till it has doubled in size in a warm oven.
8. In a separate bowl, combine the spinach, salt, feta, marjoram, and pepper.
9. On a floured surface, roll out the dough into a coarse rectangle measuring 12 x 16 inches. 1Cover the dough with the spinach mixture, leaving a 12-inch border around the borders. 1Roll the dough firmly into a log, beginning on the longer side, and squeeze to seal the edge.
10. Place this log on baking parchment and cut it into 16 equal pieces. Using a serrated knife may be more convenient.
11. 1At 380°F, preheat the oven.
12. 1The rolls should then be baked for 18 to 20 minutes or until lightly browned. 1Allow the rolls to cool slightly before serving.

Scary Strawberry Snacks

Cooking time: 0 minutes

Preparation time: 20 minutes

Servings: 1

Per serving: Calories 48, Total fat 3g, Protein 1g, Carbs 8g

Ingredients:

- 50 ml of Greek yogurt
- 16 strawberries
- 2 teaspoons of orange food coloring
- 100 g of dark chocolate, minimum
- 85% of cacao
- A cocktail stick

Instructions:

Follow the instructions below to make scary strawberry snacks.

1. In a bowl set on a pot of boiling water, melt the chocolate, occasionally stirring, until smooth. Drop the strawberries in to the chocolate mixture with care.
2. Chill the strawberries for around 20 minutes before serving. Combine the yogurt and the orange food coloring.
3. Draw on your spooky pumpkin faces with a cocktail stick dipped in orange yogurt mixture.

Cabbage and Chicken Wontons

Cooking time: 10 minutes

Preparation time: 20 minutes

Servings: 16

Per serving: Calories 130, Total fat 4g, Protein 1g, Carbs 20.8g

Ingredients:

For the Filling:

- 200 g of minced chicken breast
- 1/2 tablespoon of oyster sauce
- 50 g of pak choi
- 1 teaspoon of stevia
- 50 g of white cabbage
- 15 g of corn flour
- 16 wonton wrappers
- 50 g of drained water chestnuts
- Salt & white pepper
- 50 g of bean sprouts
- 20 g of finely chopped chives
- 1 teaspoon of sesame oil
- 1 tablespoon of light soy sauce

For the Egg wash:
- 1 teaspoon of water
- 1 egg
- For the Dipping sauce:
- 1 teaspoon of soy sauce dark
- 4 tablespoons of light soy sauce

Instructions:

Follow the instructions below to make cabbage and chicken wontons.

1. Using a food processor, puree the pak choi, water chestnuts, cabbage, & bean sprouts. You don't want to form a paste, so make sure the mix has a crunchy texture.
2. Add the chicken to the mixture in a large-sized mixing dish.
3. After that, stir in the chives, corn flour, sesame oil, salt, oyster sauce, soy sauce, stevia, and pepper.
4. Spread a wonton wrapper evenly on the palms of your hand or on greaseproof paper that has been lightly floured.
5. In the middle of the wrapper, place a teaspoon of the mixture. To produce an egg wash, whisk together the egg with the water.
6. Brush the four corners of the wonton with your finger dipped in egg wash or water. Bend the wonton halfway from one corner to the other, forming a triangle.
7. Make sure the wonton is completely sealed, with no air bubbles or holes.
8. To produce the wonton shape, compress together the larger two triangular points.
9. Deep-fried the wontons in heated oil for 2 to 3 minutes, occasionally flipping, until golden brown.
10. 1Remove the wontons from the pan and pour any excess oil onto kitchen paper. 1You could also steam the dumplings for a few minutes.
11. 1To create the dipping sauce, whisk together the soy sauces & salt. 1Enjoy the wontons with the sauce while they're still hot!

Crunchy Bleu Cheese and Balsamic Veggie Pocket

Cooking time: 0 minutes

Preparation time: 10 minutes

Servings: 1 pocket

Per serving: Calories 167, Total fat 3g, Protein 6g, Carbs 29g

Ingredients:

- 1/4 cup of purple cabbage shredded
- 1 tablespoon of cucumber finely diced
- 1/2 six-inch diameter pita pocket whole wheat
- 1 tablespoon of bleu cheese crumbled
- 1 leaf of green leaf lettuce
- 2 teaspoons of balsamic vinaigrette commercial lite
- 1 canned of quartered whole artichoke heart
- 2 tablespoons of tomato finely chopped
- 2 teaspoons of purple onion finely diced

Instructions:

Follow the instructions below to make crunchy bleu cheese and balsamic veggie pocket.

1. Before filling the pita pocket, wrap it with foil or plastic wrap to stop the pocket from breaking when stuffing.
2. Fill lettuce leaf with cabbage, cucumber, artichoke, onion, and tomato, then close the pocket.
3. Drizzle with vinaigrette & sprinkle with bleu cheese.

Easy Severed Fingers

Cooking time: 10 minutes

Preparation time: 5 minutes

Servings: 4

Per serving: Calories 33, Total fat 2g, Protein 5g, Carbs 3g

Ingredients:

- 2 tablespoons of tomato sauce
- 8 pork hotdogs

Instructions:

Follow the instructions below to make easy severed fingers.

1. Rinse the hotdogs and cook them for 4 minutes in a pot of simmering water.
2. Allow cooling after cooking.
3. To make the shape of a fingernail, slice a small piece of skin off the rounded edges of the hotdogs.
4. Then, in the center of the hotdog, cut horizontal lines to replicate the creases on your finger joints.
5. To resemble blood put the hotdogs on a platter and cover them with tomato sauce.

Tasty Eggplant Rolls Roasted

Cooking time: 20 minutes

Preparation time: 10 minutes

Servings: 8 servings16 rolls

Per serving: Calories 77, Total fat 3g, Protein 3g, Carbs 12g

Ingredients:

- 2 tablespoons of fresh lemon juice
- 1 minced green onion
- 4 tablespoons 2 oz. of cream cheese fat-free
- 1 minced clove of garlic
- 1/8 teaspoon of black pepper
- 2 medium-sized eggplants 3/4 pound each
- 1 cup of meatless pasta sauce
- 1 teaspoon of olive oil
- 16 stemmed fresh spinach leaves
- 2 tablespoons of sour cream fat-free
- 4 sun-dried tomatoes packed in oil, drained, rinsed, & minced
- 1/4 teaspoon of dried oregano

Instructions:

Follow the instructions below to make tasty eggplant rolls roasted.

1. At 450°F, preheat the oven. Set aside 2 nonstick baking trays that have been sprayed with nonstick cooking spray. Trim the ends off the eggplants. Cut eggplants into 1/4-inch thick slices lengthwise. Outer slices, which are mostly skin, should be discarded it will make around 16 slices total. Arrange the slices in a single layer on the baking sheets that have been prepared.
2. In a small-sized dish, combine the lemon juice & olive oil; lightly brush both sides of the eggplant pieces. Bake for

around 20 minutes, flipping once or until golden brown. Place eggplant slices on a dish to cool.

3. In a small-sized mixing bowl, combine cream cheese, sour cream, oregano, green onion, sun- dried tomatoes, garlic, and pepper.

4. Evenly spread 1 teaspoon of cream cheese mixture on each eggplant slice. Place one spinach leaf on top of the other, leaving a 1/2-inch border. Begin rolling from the tiny end. Place the rolls on a serving plate, seam side down. Cover and chill for up to 2 days if making ahead. Before serving, allow it cool to room temperature. Serve with the warmed pasta sauce before serving.

Melon and Parma Ham Balls

Cooking time: 0 minutes

Preparation time: 10 minutes

Servings: 4

Per serving: Calories 107, Total fat 2g, Protein 1g, Carbs 27g

Ingredients:

- Cocktail sticks
- 200 g of Parma ham
- 1 melon

Instructions:

Follow the instructions below to make melon and Parma ham balls. Scrape the seeds out of the melon by cutting them in half.

1. Using a melon cutter, remove the seeds and chop out portions of the melon.
2. Insert the melon balls onto the cocktail sticks, add small rolled-up pieces of Parma ham, more melon balls, and more ham slices until the cocktail stick is full.

Delicious Buffalo Chicken

Cooking time: 20 minutes

Preparation time: 10 minutes

Servings: 42 pieces

Per serving: Calories 154, Total fat 6g, Protein 24g, Carbs 1g

Ingredients:

- 2 teaspoons of dried parsley
- Cooking spray
- 1/2 cup of red hot sauce
- Celery sticks
- 1 pound of cooked chicken breasts, make bite-size chunks
- Ranch or blue cheese salad dressing low-fat
- 3 tablespoons of melted margarine low-fat
- 1/4 teaspoon of garlic powder

Instructions:

Follow the instructions below to make delicious buffalo chicken.

1. At 350°F, preheat the oven. Put chicken bites in a baking dish that has been sprayed with cooking spray.
2. Combine the Red Hot sauce, parsley, margarine, and garlic powder in a mixing dish.
3. Pour over the chicken in an equal layer.
4. You can keep the combined chicken & sauce in the refrigerator until ready to heat & serve.
5. Bake for around 20 minutes. Place every piece of chicken on a serving platter with a toothpick.
6. Toss with celery sticks & salad dressing before serving.

Festive Pesto Mini Chicken Kebabs

Cooking time: 10 minutes

Preparation time: 10 minutes

Servings: 8

Per serving: Calories 59, Total fat 6g, Protein 3g, Carbs 1g

Ingredients:

- 2 tablespoons of agave nectar
- 400 g of chicken breasts
- 2 chicken breasts, halved with each half slice into
- 12 long strips
- Oil for the backing tray
- 60 g of green pesto
- 24 small wooden or metal skewers

Instructions:

Follow the instructions below to make a festive pesto mini chicken kebabs.

1. At 350°F, preheat the oven.
2. Combine the pesto, chicken, and agave nectar.
3. Skewer the meat onto the skewer & place them on a lightly greased baking pan in the preheated oven.
4. Bake for around 8 minutes or until the meat is thoroughly cooked. Enjoy! Serve on a plate.

Tempting Salmon Seaweed Wraps

Cooking time: 0 minutes

Preparation time: 20 minutes

Servings: 2

Per serving: Calories 188, Total fat 7g, Protein 22g, Carbs 13g

Ingredients:

- 2 teaspoons of fresh lemon juice
- 1 6-ounces can of drained salmon
- 3 whole romaine lettuce leaves
- 1/2 ripe avocado
- 1/4 teaspoon of salt
- 1/2 cup of a diced small cucumber
- 1/2 cup of diced small celery
- 1/2 cup of red pepper thinly cut into 2-inch strips
- Pepper to taste
- 1/2 cup of daikon radish, diced small
- 3 nori sheets typically for making sushi

Instructions:

Follow the instructions below to make tempting salmon seaweed wraps.

1. Mash the salmon with a fork in a large-sized mixing dish, including the bones. Remove the avocado from the skin with a spoon & mix it into the salmon. Continue mashing.
2. Add diced celery & daikon to the mix. Toss in the lemon juice and season with salt and black pepper to taste. Blend thoroughly.
3. On a flat plate or chopping board, place one nori sheet. One romaine lettuce leaf should be placed on top of the nori sheet toward one of the edges.

4. Spread 1/3 cup of the salmon mixture onto the lettuce leaf and spread it out evenly. Cucumber dice & red pepper sticks go on top.
5. Wrap the nori sheet tightly across the lettuce & filling using your hands. Using a little water, wet the nori's edge to seal the wrap.

Cocktail Nuts with Maple Glazed

Cooking time: 10 minutes

Preparation time: 10 minutes

Servings: 6

Per serving: Calories 240, Total fat 22g, Protein 3g, Carbs 8g

Ingredients:

- 50 g of cashews
- 2 teaspoons of Stevia
- 100 g cup of almonds
- 2 teaspoons of maple syrup
- 50 g of pecans
- Salt to taste
- 50 g of peanuts
- 2 tablespoons of melted butter

Instructions:

Follow the instructions below to make cocktail nuts with maple glazed. At 350°F, preheat the oven.

1. Using baking parchment, line a baking tray.
2. In a large-sized mixing dish, combine all of the nuts. Combine the maple syrup, melted butter, and Stevia in a dish. Season with salt and add to the nut mixture.
3. Bake for around 10 minutes, tossing every few minutes on the baking tray.
4. Remove from the oven and allow to cool before serving!

Pigs Wrapped in Blankets

Cooking time: 25 minutes

Preparation time: 5 minutes

Servings: 12

Per serving: Calories 69, Total fat 3g, Protein 3g, Carbs 1g

Ingredients:

- 6 rashes of English bacon unsmoked
- 1 pack of premium pork chipolatas mostly contains around 12 cocktail sausages

Instructions:

Follow the instructions below to make pigs wrapped in blankets. At 370°F, preheat the oven.

1. Next, half each rasher of bacon & lengthen each one without splitting it, then roll the bacon in a spiral across the body of the sausage.
2. Roast for around 20 to 25 minutes, flipping after 15 minutes to ensure that the sausage is properly cooked.
3. Ensure that the sausage is heated completely & that no pink parts remain before serving.

Delicious Watercress with Pancetta

Cooking time: 20 minutes

Preparation time: 10 minutes

Servings: 4

Per serving: Calories 108, Total fat 3g, Protein 8g, Carbs 6g

Ingredients:

- 1 small potato, diced, peeled, and washed
- 150g of watercress
- 1l of vegetable stock
- 2 rashers of pancetta or the other bacon
- 1 tablespoon of olive oil
- 20 g of butter
- 2 finely chopped and peeled garlic cloves

Instructions:

Follow the instructions below to make delicious watercress with pancetta.

1. Place the onions in a pan with butter & olive oil and sauté on medium flame till the onions soften for about 4 minutes.
2. Add the celeriac, stock, & garlic with the onion combination.
3. Cook, occasionally stirring, for about 10 minutes, or until the potatoes are softened. Blend the soup until it reaches a smooth consistency.
4. Lightly fry the pancetta and cut it into small pieces. Toss in the watercress and stir to combine.
5. Take the soup from the stove & puree it until it has a creamy texture. Before serving, divide into four dishes and top with pancetta!

Greek-Style Shrimps

Cooking time: 25 minutes

Preparation time: 5 minutes

Servings: 5

Per serving: Calories 189, Total fat 5g, Protein 21g, Carbs 15g

Ingredients:

- 1/4 cup of fresh parsley chopped
- 1 cup of chicken broth
- 1 tablespoon of olive oil
- 1/4 cup of Mizithra cheese grated
- 1/2 teaspoon of stevia
- 1 pound of medium-size cooked shrimp, peeled & deveined
- 1 minced clove of garlic
- 1 chopped large onion
- 11/2 pounds of peeled & chopped Roma tomatoes

Instructions:

Follow the instructions below to make Greek-style shrimps.

1. In a large-sized nonstick skillet, heat the oil on medium flame. Add the onion and cook for 3 to 4 minutes, or until tender. Combine the parsley, garlic, & stevia. Cook, uncovered, until the tomatoes are softened, and the liquid has evaporated, approximately 5 minutes; stir regularly. Cook, occasionally stirring, until the liquid has evaporated, about 10 minutes. Cook, stirring periodically, for 2 to 3 minutes, or till shrimp are well heated. Top with cheese & move to a serving dish. Serve over brown rice that has been cooked.

Tasty Baba Ghanoush Eggplant Dip

Cooking time: 20 minutes

Preparation time: 10 minutes

Servings: 2 1/3 cups

Per serving: Calories 74, Total fat 5g, Protein 2g, Carbs 7g

Ingredients:

- 2 minced cloves of garlic
- 1 tablespoon of minced fresh parsley
- 1 eggplant large
- 3 tablespoons of fresh lemon juice
- 1 teaspoon of olive oil
- 2 tablespoons of tahini paste
- 1/2 teaspoon of cayenne pepper

Instructions:

Follow the instructions below to make tasty baba ghanoush eggplant dip.

1. At 400°F, preheat the oven. Using a knife, cut the eggplant in 1/2 lengthwise. Place it cut side down on a baking pan. Bake for around 20 minutes in a hot oven, or until the skin is black and the eggplant is tender & cooked through. Meanwhile, in a small-sized mixing dish, combine the tahini, garlic, and lemon juice.

2. Remove the eggplant halves from the oven when they are done & run cold water onto them for one minute. Drain the water and allow it to cool somewhat. The skin should be removed. Slice the eggplant and combine it with the tahini mixture in a mixing bowl.

3. To create a lumpy dip, mash the eggplant also with the remaining ingredients. Pour the olive oil on the top of the

sauce and sprinkle with parsley & cayenne pepper. Chill until ready to serve. Represent with pita triangles on the side.

Delicious Cheesy Polenta with Mushrooms

Cooking time: 20 minutes

Preparation time: 10 minutes

Servings: 5

Per serving: Calories 185, Total fat 7g, Protein 9g, Carbs 21g

Ingredients:

- 20 button mushrooms
- 500 g of ready-made polenta
- 100 ml of milk semi-skimmed
- 2 tablespoons of butter
- 100 g of peeled & finely chopped onions
- 100 ml of single cream
- 2 peeled & finely chopped cloves of garlic

Instructions:

Follow the instructions below to make delicious cheesy polenta with mushrooms. At 390°F, preheat the oven.

1. In a medium-sized saucepan, melt the butter.
2. In a small amount of butter, soften the onions for a few minutes. Cook for a few minutes after adding the mushrooms & garlic.
3. Remove the pan from the stove.
4. Return the onion mixture to the burner after carefully adding the cream & milk. Bake for around 15 minutes, depending on the number of servings.
5. Once the polenta is ready, warm the sauce through and serve.

Soups And Stews Recipes

Tasty Thai Green Soup

Cooking time: 15 minutes

Preparation time: 10 minutes

Servings: 4

Per serving: Calories 205, Total fat 12g, Protein 9g, Carbs 19g

Ingredients:

- 3 finely chopped garlic cloves
- Chopped broccoli head
- 120 g of green peas
- 50 ml of olive oil
- 120 g of chopped green beans
- 100 g of spinach leaves
- Finely chopped onion
- 1 roughly chopped courgette
- 120g of asparagus, trimmed & cut into inch long pieces
- 1 finely chopped celery stick
- 1.5 l of vegetable stock

Instructions:

Follow the instructions below to make tasty Thai green soup.

1. In a skillet, heat the olive oil & sauté the garlic, onion, and celery until slightly browned. Cook for around 5 minutes after adding the courgette & broccoli.
2. Pour in the stock and bring the whole thing to a boil.
3. Mix in the asparagus, green beans, peas, and spinach after a few minutes of simmering. Cook for another 5 minutes, or till the vegetables are fully cooked.
4. Salt and black pepper to taste.
5. Blend everything together in a blender & serve!

Tofu Soup Sweet and Sour

Cooking time: 15 minutes

Preparation time: 5 minutes

Servings: 4

Per serving: Calories 63, Total fat 1g, Protein 3g, Carbs 9g

Ingredients:

- 1carrot, juliennes cut
- 2 l of vegetable stock
- 175g of diced tofu
- 2 teaspoons of stevia
- 30 g of baby spinach
- 1/2 tablespoon of red Thai curry paste
- 1 1/2 tablespoons of soy sauce
- 1/2 lime juice

Instructions:

Follow the instructions below to make tofu soup sweet and sour.

1. In a large-sized pan, heat the vegetable stock & add the red curry paste. On a medium flame, constantly stir till the paste has fully dissolved.
2. Simmer for 5 minutes after adding the stevia, soy sauce, and carrots. Pour the hot soup over the tofu in four dishes.
3. Serve with spinach as a garnish.

Delicious Cajun Stew

Cooking time: 25 minutes

Preparation time: 5 minutes

Servings: 4

Per serving: Calories 199, Total fat 6g, Protein 14g, Carbs 24g

Ingredients:

- 1chopped onion
- 22-ounce of turkey or chicken andouille sausage links, cut into thick 1/4-inch pieces
- 1 minced clove of garlic
- 2 cups of frozen sliced okra
- 1/4 teaspoon of salt
- 1 teaspoon of olive oil
- 1/8 teaspoon of dried thyme
- 1 cup of chicken broth low-sodium
- 1/4 teaspoon of red pepper flakes
- 1 chopped stalk of celery
- 1 boneless & skinless chicken thigh around
- 4 ounces, chopped into bite-size chunks
- 1 can around 14 ounces of tomatoes no-salt-added diced
- 1 cup of brown rice cooked
- 1/8 teaspoon of black pepper

Instructions:

Follow the instructions below to make delicious Cajun stew.

1. In a large-sized saucepan, heat the oil at medium-high flame. Cook and stir for 3 minutes after adding the celery, onion, and garlic. Add turkey and chicken, cook and stir for 2 minutes, or until chicken & turkey sausage are browned on all sides. Stir in the broth to scrape off any browned bits.

2. In a saucepan, combine tomatoes, okra, black pepper, rice, red pepper flakes, salt, and thyme. Bring the mixture to a boil. Reduce to a low flame setting, cover, and simmer for 10 minutes.

Tasty Braised Pork Stew

Cooking time: 25 minutes

Preparation time: 5 minutes

Servings: 4

Per serving: Calories 250, Total fat 8g, Protein 26g, Carbs 16g

Ingredients:

- 5 tablespoons of all-purpose flour, divided
- 1/2 teaspoon of salt
- 16 ounces of frozen vegetables assorted
- 2 teaspoons of stone-ground mustard
- 1 pound of pork tenderloin, chopped into 1-inch cubes
- 2 tablespoons of water
- 1/2 teaspoon of pepper
- 1-1/2 cups of chicken broth reduced-sodium
- 1 tablespoon of olive oil
- 1 teaspoon of dried thyme
- 2 minced garlic cloves

Instructions:

Follow the instructions below to make tasty braised pork stew.

1. Season pork with salt and black pepper, then toss with 3 tablespoons flour to coat. Heat the oil in a large-sized skillet on medium flame. Pork should be browned. If required, drain. Combine the veggies, broth, mustard, garlic, and thyme. Bring the mixture to a boil. Reduce flame to low; cover & cook for 10 to 15 minutes, or until pork and veggies are cooked.
2. Combine the remaining flour & water in a small-sized dish until smooth; mix into the stew. Return them to a boil, frequently stirring, for 1 to 2 minutes, or until the sauce has thickened.

Kidney and Black Bean Soup

Cooking time: 25 minutes

Preparation time: 5 minutes

Servings: 2

Per serving: Calories 201, Total fat 3g, Protein 4g, Carbs 23g

Ingredients:
- 3 finely chopped cloves of garlic
- 175 g of rinsed & drained tinned black beans
- 1 finely chopped carrot
- 175 g of rinsed & drained tinned kidney beans
- 1 teaspoon of freshly ground pepper
- 2 l of vegetable stock
- 2 teaspoons of oregano
- 1 tablespoon of olive oil
- 1 finely chopped onion
- 1 teaspoon of sea salt
- 1finely chopped stalk of celery

Instructions:

Follow the instructions below to make kidney and black bean soup.

1. In a pot of freshwater, bring the two varieties of beans to a boil and then reduce to a low flame for 10 minutes. After that, drain.
2. On medium heat, heat the olive oil.
3. The onions should then be fried for almost 5 minutes. Combine the oregano, vegetables, and salt and black pepper. Add the beans & vegetable stock after that.
4. Cook for another 10 minutes, covered.
5. You may eat the soup as is or purée half of it in a blender. Serve with parsley as a garnish and enjoy!

Tempting Tomato Soup

Cooking time: 25 minutes

Preparation time: 5 minutes

Servings: 2

Per serving: Calories 315, Total fat 11g, Protein 2g, Carbs 35g

Ingredients:

- 2 celery sticks
- 2 teaspoons of tomato purée
- 1-25 kg of ripe tomatoes
- 2 liters of hot vegetable stock
- 2 cloves of garlic
- 2 bay leaves
- 1onion medium
- Fresh basil for garnishing
- 1 carrot large
- 2 tablespoons of olive oil

Instructions:

Follow the instructions below to make tempting tomato soup.

1. To begin, clean the tomatoes and quarter them, removing any hard cores with a knife.
2. Peel and chop the garlic, onion, and carrot into small pieces. Cut the celery into pieces that are about the same size.
3. In a large-sized saucepan, heat the olive oil on a low flame. Put the garlic, onion, carrots, & celery.
4. Cook, occasionally stirring, for around 5 minutes, or until the veggies are softened.
5. Stir the tomatoes, tomato purée, & black pepper into the vegetables. Stir the bay leaves and continue to cook over a low flame for about 5 minutes, or until everything in the pan has shrunk and the juices are running.

6. Stir constantly until all of the vegetables are well combined. Pour the heated stock in slowly.
7. Turn the flame to high and allow the mixture to bubble for a few minutes before lowering the flame to low.
8. Replace the cap and simmer for another 15 minutes on low heat, stirring occasionally. 1When the soup is done, turn off the heat, give it a thorough stir, and discard all the bay leaves. 1Blend the ingredients until smooth by slowly pouring them into a blender.
9. 1With a dusting of broken basil leaves on top, serve.

Lentil Zesty Soup

Cooking time: 25 minutes

Preparation time: 5 minutes

Servings: 2

Per serving: Calories 174, Total fat 0.3g, Protein 3g, Carbs 23g

Ingredients:

- 3 tablespoons of red lentils or puy
- 1 roughly chopped onion
- 1 tablespoon of olive oil
- 300 ml of vegetable stock
- 1 peeled & grated large carrot
- A pinch of chili flakes optional
- 1 lime juice & zest
- 1 teaspoon of cumin seeds
- 1 x 400 g tin of chopped tomatoes

Instructions:

Follow the instructions below to make lentil zesty soup.

1. In a small amount of oil, soften the onion & carrot for around 4 minutes. Sprinkle the chili flakes & cumin seeds.
2. After a minute, add the tomato, lentils, and stock and cook for another minute. Cook, occasionally stirring, for 10 to 15 minutes, or till the lentils are tender. To achieve a creamy consistency, pulse rapidly with a stick blender.
3. Before serving, add the lime zest and juice.

Simple Mushroom Soup

Cooking time: 25 minutes

Preparation time: 5 minutes

Servings: 2

Per serving: Calories 314, Total fat 46g, Protein 15g, Carbs 25g

Ingredients:

- 200 g of Portobello mushrooms
- 3 cloves of garlic
- 1litre of chicken or vegetable stock
- Bunch of fresh thyme
- 200 g of dried porcini mushrooms
- Fresh parsley chopped
- 3 tablespoons of olive oil
- 10 g of freshly ground black pepper
- 200 g of chestnut mushrooms
- Sea salt
- 1 onion medium
- 1 lemon juice

Instructions:

Follow the instructions below to make simple mushroom soup.

1. Immerse the dried porcini mushrooms for around 30 minutes in water or as directed on the package.
2. Cut the onion & mushrooms into tiny pieces. In a large-sized skillet, warm 1 tablespoon of olive oil and add the crushed garlic and chopped onion.
3. Allow 5 minutes for the mixture to simmer down.
4. Cook for another 5 minutes till the mushroom release their juices, then place the mushrooms in the pan & top with the leftover olive oil.

5. Remove the fresh thyme stalks & combine with the freshly ground black pepper & stock. Cook for 15 minutes, covered.
6. Blend with a stick blender until the texture is semi-smooth. Squeeze in some lemon juice.
7. Taste for seasoning and season with more salt and black pepper if necessary. Serve with chopped parsley on top.

Quick and Tasty White Bean Soup

Cooking time: 25 minutes

Preparation time: 5 minutes

Servings: 6

Per serving: Calories 162, Total fat 3g, Protein 9g, Carbs 28g

Ingredients:

- 3 chopped stalks of celery
- 4 cups of vegetable stock or water
- 1 cup of dried white beans such as great northern, navy, or cannellini, soaked overnight
- 1 can of diced tomatoes 14 ounces
- 1 tablespoon of olive oil
- Freshly shredded Parmesan cheese optional
- 1 chopped large onion
- Salt to taste
- 1/2 teaspoon of dried sage
- Freshly ground pepper
- 1to 2 cups of fresh spinach chopped
- Basil pesto optional

Instructions:

Follow the instructions below to make quick and tasty white bean soup.

1. Beans should be drained. In a pressure cooker, heat the oil and add the celery, drained beans, onion, and a couple of pinches of fresh pepper.
2. Cook for around 5 minutes until the veggies and beans are aromatic. Add the stock or water, as well as the sage.
3. Secure the cover and raise the pressure to high.
4. The cooking time is 20 minutes.
5. Wait for natural pressure release after turning off the flame.

6. Remove the cover and toss in the tomatoes and spinach.
7. Cook until the spinach is tender.
8. Season with salt and freshly ground black pepper.
9. Serve with a dollop of basil pesto or freshly grated Parmesan cheese.

Spinach, Chicken and Wild Rice Soup

Cooking time: 20 minutes

Preparation time: 5 minutes

Servings: 6 to 7

Per serving: Calories 256, Total fat 7g, Protein 22g, Carbs 28g

Ingredients:

- 2 cups of baby spinach coarsely chopped
- 1/4 teaspoon of dried sage
- 1 can of reduced-sodium chicken broth about
- 14 ounces 2 cups of wild rice cooked
- 1/2 cup of half-and-half fat-free or fat-free skim milk
- 1 3/4 cups of carrots chopped
- 1 teaspoon of dried thyme
- 2 cans of reduced-fat & reduced-sodium condensed cream of chicken soup, undiluted about 10 3/4 ounces each
- 1/4 teaspoon of black pepper
- 1 1/2 cups of cooked chicken chopped

Instructions:

Follow the instructions below to make spinach, chicken and wild rice soup.

1. In a large-sized saucepan on a medium-high flame, bring the broth to a boil. Cook for 10 minutes after adding the carrots.
2. Bring the soup, rice, sage, thyme, and pepper to a boil in a saucepan. Cook & stir for 2 minutes, or until chicken, spinach, and half-and-half are heated thoroughly.

Tasty Butternut Bisque

Cooking time: 25 minutes

Preparation time: 5 minutes

Servings: 6

Per serving: Calories 79, Total fat 1g, Protein 5g, Carbs 14g

Ingredients:

- 1 butternut squash medium around 1 1/2 pounds, make 1/2-inch pieces
- 1/8 teaspoon of white pepper
- 1 teaspoon of margarine
- 1/2 teaspoon of ground nutmeg
- 1 large coarsely chopped onion
- 2 cans of reduced-sodium chicken broth around 14 ounces each, divided
- Plain yogurt non-fat & chopped chives optional

Instructions:

Follow the instructions below to make tasty butternut bisque.

1. In a large-sized saucepan, melt margarine on medium flame. Cook and stir for 3 minutes after adding the onion. Bring one can of broth with squash to a boil on high flame. Reduce to a low heat setting, cover, and cook for 20 minutes, or until the squash is very soft.
2. In a blender, puree the soup in batches, returning the pureed soup to the saucepan with each batch. Alternatively, a hand-held immersion blender can be used. Combine the leftover can of broth, nutmeg, & black pepper in a large-sized bowl. Cook for 5 minutes, uncovered, stirring periodically.

Moroccan Vegetable and Lentil Soup

Cooking time: 25 minutes

Preparation time: 5 minutes

Servings: 6

Per serving: Calories 131, Total fat 3g, Protein 8g, Carbs 20g

Ingredients:

- 4 minced cloves of garlic
- 1 1/2 teaspoons of ground cumin
- 1 tablespoon of olive oil
- 1/2 teaspoon of black pepper
- 1/2 cup of celery chopped
- 1 cup of plum tomatoes chopped
- 1 1/2 teaspoons of ground coriander
- 1 cup of onion chopped
- 1 chopped yellow squash
- 1/4 cup of fresh cilantro or basil chopped
- 1/2 cup of rinsed & sorted dried lentils
- 1/2 cup of fresh Italian parsley chopped
- 1/2 teaspoon of ground cinnamon
- 1container of low-sodium vegetable broth 32 ounces
- 1/2 cup of sun-dried tomatoes chopped not packed in oil
- 1/2 cup of green bell pepper chopped

Instructions:

Follow the instructions below to make Moroccan vegetable and lentil soup.

1. In a medium-sized saucepan, heat the oil at medium-high flame. Add the garlic and onions and simmer, frequently stirring, for 2 minutes, or until the onion is soft. Cook for 2 minutes after adding the lentils, cinnamon, coriander, cumin, and black pepper. Bring to a boil with the celery, broth, and

sun-dried tomatoes. Reduce to medium-low flame, cover, and cook for 15 minutes.

2. Cook for 10 minutes, or until lentils are cooked, stirring in squash & bell pepper. Just before serving, garnish with parsley, plum tomatoes, and cilantro.

Parsnip Soup Spicy

Cooking time: 25 minutes

Preparation time: 5 minutes

Servings: 6

Per serving: Calories 161, Total fat 1g, Protein 4g, Carbs 38g

Ingredients:

- 700 g of parsnips
- 2 teaspoons of cumin seeds
- 4 cloves of finely chopped garlic
- Fresh parsley to garnish
- 1 potato medium
- 1/2 tablespoon of ground ginger
- Finely chopped onion
- 1 liter of vegetable stock
- 1 1/2 teaspoon of ground turmeric
- 1 1/2 teaspoons of ground coriander
- 1 teaspoon of black mustard seeds
- 1 tablespoon of fresh lemon juice
- 275 ml of low-fat natural yogurt
- Freshly ground nutmeg to garnish

Instructions:

Follow the instructions below to make parsnip soup spicy.

1. In a pan with 50ml of water, combine the parsnips, potato, and onion.
2. Bring the water to a boil, then reduce the flame to low and simmer for the next 10 minutes. Combine the spices, garlic, ginger, and lemon juice.
3. Cook for another 2 minutes, stirring constantly. Pour the stock in.

4. Put the mixture to a boil, then reduce to low heat and cook for about 10 minutes. Blend the contents in a blender and return them to the pan.
5. Stir in the yogurt, season with coriander, & garnish with fresh parsley and grated nutmeg before serving.

Festive-Style Spinach Soup

Cooking time: 25 minutes

Preparation time: 5 minutes

Servings: 6

Per serving: Calories 285, Total fat 12g, Protein 3g, Carbs 29g

Ingredients:

- 3 finely chopped garlic cloves
- 900 ml of milk
- 75 g of butter
- Ground nutmeg, to taste
- 1 finely chopped large onion
- 625 g of vegetable stock
- 1lemon zest and juice
- 2 peeled & diced medium potatoes
- 5 tablespoons of double cream, to serve
- 625g of fresh spinach, washed if necessary & roughly chopped

Instructions:

Follow the instructions below to make festive-style spinach soup.

1. Allow the butter to melt slowly in a big, covered saucepan at low flame.
2. After that, mix the onion & garlic and cook for 5-6 minutes, or until softened. Mix in the potato & simmer for another minute.
3. Put in the stock & continue to cook for another 8-10 minutes, or till the potato is tender. Mix in 1/2 of the spinach as well as the lemon zest after adding the milk.
4. Cover and cook for 10 minutes, or till the spinach has wilted fully. Allow 5 minutes for the soup to cool.
5. In a blender, puree the soup.

6. To maintain the soup bright & fresh-tasting, add the remaining spinach. Sprinkle with salt, pepper, & nutmeg after blending the soup till silky smooth.
7. 1To serve, reheat the soup until it's hot, then spoon it into bowls with a swirl of double cream.

Yummy Butternut Squash Soup

Cooking time: 25 minutes

Preparation time: 5 minutes

Servings: 4

Per serving: Calories 73, Total fat 0.1g, Protein 2g, Carbs 13g

Ingredients:

- 1 finely chopped small onion
- 750 ml of vegetable stock
- 400 g of peeled and diced butternut squash
- 100 ml of skimmed milk
- 1 peeled and diced carrot
- 1 finely chopped celery stalk
- 2 finely chopped garlic cloves
- Salt & freshly ground pepper

Instructions:

Follow the instructions below to make yummy butternut squash soup.

1. In a large-sized pot, bring the butternut squash, carrot, garlic, celery, onion, and vegetable stock to a boil.
2. Reduce the flame to low and cook for about 25 minutes, or until the squash is tender. In a blender, purée the soup by adding the milk to the mixture.
3. Season with salt and black pepper, and enjoy!

Asparagus Soup Spicy

Cooking time: 25 minutes

Preparation time: 5 minutes

Servings: 4

Per serving: Calories 254, Total fat 12g, Protein 6g, Carbs 14g

Ingredients:

- 400 ml of half-fat coconut milk
- 300 g of asparagus
- 1tablespoon of sesame oil
- 1 diced shallot
- 400 ml of slightly salted water
- Pinch of salt
- 2 finely chopped garlic cloves
- 1/4 teaspoon of ground white pepper
- 1 tablespoon of light soy sauce

Instructions:

Follow the instructions below to make asparagus soup spicy.

1. In a saucepan, place the asparagus & cover it with lightly salted water.
2. Bring to a boil, reduce to a low flame and cook for 3 minutes with the asparagus spears. Rinse the asparagus and liquidize it in 400ml of the same water that was used to boil it. In a medium-sized saucepan, heat the sesame oil on medium flame.
3. Sauté for 1 minute with the shallot, garlic, and pepper.
4. Bring the liquidized asparagus to a boil with the rest of the ingredients.
5. After that, pour the coconut milk and cook for 2 minutes before adding the soy sauce. Now the food is ready to eat.

6. Season with salt and black pepper to taste, then top with
   watercress.

Thai Mixed Veg and Coconut Soup

Cooking time: 15 minutes

Preparation time: 5 minutes

Servings: 4

Per serving: Calories 215, Total fat 18g, Protein 6g, Carbs 13g

Ingredients:
- 2 tablespoons of finely chopped ginger
- 800 ml of coconut milk half-fat
- 1 tablespoon of vegetable oil
- 300 ml of water
- 600 g of stir-fry vegetables
- 2 minced garlic cloves
- Fresh coriander to garnish
- 2 teaspoons of vegetarian green
- Thai paste
- 1 red chili

Instructions:

Follow the instructions below to make Thai mixed veg and coconut soup. In a wok, warm the vegetable oil on medium flame.

1. In a wok, stir-fry the vegetables for 3 minutes.
2. Cook for a minute after adding the garlic, ginger, & chili.
3. In a bowl, combine the green Thai paste, coconut milk with water. Pour the liquid mixture over the veggies in the pan.
4. Put the mixture to a boil, covered in the wok.
5. Cook for an additional 2 minutes before dividing the soup into 4 bowls. Serve with coriander as a garnish.

Delicious Sweetcorn Soup

Cooking time: 20 minutes

Preparation time: 5 minutes

Servings: 4

Per serving: Calories 214, Total fat 14g, Protein 4g, Carbs 19g

Ingredients:

- 1 finely sliced onion
- 180 g of diced celeriac
- Salt & freshly ground black pepper
- 30 g of butter
- 220 g of tinned sweetcorn
- 2 tablespoons of olive oil
- 2 finely chopped garlic cloves
- 800 ml of vegetable stock, made out of two vegetable stock cubes
- Coriander for garnish

Instructions:

Follow the instructions below to make delicious sweetcorn soup.

1. Warm the butter and olive oil in a medium-sized saucepan on medium flame until the butter has melted and the pan is hot.
2. Add the garlic, onion and celeriac and cook for 3 minutes, or until softened. Put the mixture to a boil with the vegetable stock.
3. Reduce the heat to low & cook the stock for around 6 minutes, ensuring the celeriac is fully cooked celeriac darkens once cooked.
4. Add salt and pepper, then blend until smooth in a food processor.

5. Return to the pot, add the sweetcorn and continue to simmer for another two minutes. Serve the soup in four dishes garnished with coriander.

Mushroom and Chicken Soup

Cooking time: 15 minutes

Preparation time: 5 minutes

Servings: 6

Per serving: Calories 214, Total fat 14g, Protein 4g, Carbs 19g

Ingredients:

- 1 tablespoon of low-sodium soy sauce
- 1 tablespoon of dry sherry
- 1qtr. of low-sodium chicken broth low-fat
- 1 cup of stems removed sliced mushrooms
- 1/2 lb. of boneless and skinless
- 1/2-inch chicken breasts cubed
- 1 tablespoon of minced scallions

Instructions:

Follow the instructions below to make mushroom and chicken soup.

1. In a saucepan, add all ingredients and cook everything together for around 15 minutes on medium-low flame.

Most Popular Diabetic Recipes

Toothsome Cauliflower Pizza

Cooking time: 25 minutes

Preparation time: 5 minutes

Servings: 4

Per serving: Calories 294, Total fat 17g, Protein 12g, Carbs 13g

Ingredients:

For the Pizza Base:

- 3 teaspoons of dried oregano
- Himalayan sea salt & freshly ground black pepper to season
- Whole cauliflower grated
- 3 beaten free-range eggs
- 75g of almond flour

For the Pizza topping:

- 50 g of mozzarella grated
- 1 shaved courgette, shave using a potato peeler

For the tomato sauce:

- 400 g of finely chopped tinned tomatoes
- 2 tablespoons of olive oil
- Freshly ground salt & pepper to season
- 1 small finely chopped onion
- 5 sprigs of basil, leaves picked
- 3 minced garlic cloves

Instructions:

Follow the instructions below to make toothsome cauliflower pizza.

TO MAKE THE TOMATO SAUCE:

1. Pour the oil into a skillet & heat it on medium flame. Sauté the onion & garlic for 3 to 4 minutes.

2. Place the basil, salt, tomatoes, and pepper.
3. Reduce the flame to low, cover, & cook for about 10 minutes.

TO MAKE THE BASE AND TOPPING:

1. At 400°F, preheat the oven.
2. Greaseproof paper should be used to line a baking tray.
3. Grate the cauliflower finely and combine it with the almond flour, salt, oregano, and pepper in a mixing dish.
4. Place all of the ingredients in a volcano-shaped pile, hollow out the middle, and crack the eggs into it.
5. Fold the ingredients together using your hands till a dough forms.
6. Transfer the dough to the greaseproof paper & shape it into a pizza base by hand. Make the foundation as level as possible, with the sides slightly raised, so the top does not slip off. 1In a preheated oven, bake for 10 minutes.
7. Return to the oven for another five minutes after adding the shaved courgette, tomato sauce, and grated mozzarella.
8. Now is the time to savor your meal!

Stuffed Bell Peppers with Turkey

Cooking time: 15 minutes

Preparation time: 15 minutes

Servings: 5 2 stuffed peppers

Per serving: Calories 323, Total fat 10g, Protein 40g, Carbs 20g

Ingredients:

- 2 teaspoons of ground cumin
- 5 medium green, yellow or red peppers
- 1/2 teaspoon of pepper
- 1-1/2 cups of soft bread crumbs
- 2 teaspoons of olive oil
- 1 chopped large onion
- 1-3/4 cups of cheddar-flavored lactose-free shredded
- 1 teaspoon of Italian seasoning
- 1-1/4 pounds of ground turkey extra-lean 99% lean
- 1/4 teaspoon of paprika
- 1minced garlic clove
- 1/2 teaspoon of salt
- 2 finely chopped medium tomatoes

Instructions:

Follow the instructions below to make stuffed bell peppers with turkey.

1. At 350°F, preheat the oven. Remove the seeds from the peppers by cutting them in half lengthwise. Place in a 15x10x1-inch baking pan that has been sprayed with cooking spray.
2. Warm the oil in a large-sized skillet on medium-high flame. On a medium-high flame, cook & crumble turkey alongside garlic, onion, and seasonings until flesh is no pinker, 6 to 8

minutes. Allow cooling slightly. Combine the cheese, tomatoes, and bread crumbs.

3. Fill with the turkey filling. Paprika should be sprinkled on top. Bake for around 15 minutes, uncovered until the filling is warmed through and the peppers are soft.

Tasty Corn on the Cob with Citrus Buttery Spread

Cooking time: 20 minutes

Preparation time: 5 minutes

Servings: 4

Per serving: Calories 84, Total fat 3g, Protein 2g, Carbs 15g

Ingredients:

- 2 tablespoons of reduced-fat margarine
- 1/2 teaspoon of black pepper
- 4 medium ears of corn, husks & silks removed
- 1/4 teaspoon of salt
- Nonstick cooking spray
- 1 tablespoon of parsley finely chopped
- 1/4 teaspoon of paprika
- 1 teaspoon of grated lemon peel

Instructions:

Follow the instructions below to make tasty corn on the cob with citrus buttery spread.

1. At medium, preheat the grill. Using nonstick cooking spray, coat the corn. Grill for around 18 to 20 minutes, covered, till golden brown, turning regularly.
2. Meanwhile, in a small-sized mixing dish, combine the remaining ingredients. Corn should be served with a spread.

Spiced Pineapple, Halibut and Pepper Skewers

Cooking time: 20 minutes

Preparation time: 5 minutes

Servings: 6

Per serving: Calories 84, Total fat 1g, Protein 8g, Carbs 11g

Ingredients:

- 1/2 pound of boneless & skinless halibut steak, around 1-inch thick
- 1 teaspoon of chili powder
- 1/4 teaspoon of ground cinnamon
- 1large red or green bell pepper, make 24 pieces
- 1 teaspoon of minced garlic
- 1/8 teaspoon of ground cloves
- 2 tablespoons of fresh lemon juice or lime juice
- 1/2 small pineapple, halved lengthwise, peeled, & cut into 24 pieces
- 1/2 teaspoon of ground cumin

Instructions:

Follow the instructions below to make spiced pineapple, halibut and pepper skewers.

1. In a large-sized resealable food storage bag, combine the lemon juice, cinnamon, garlic, chili powder, cumin, and cloves; knead until well combined.
2. Rinse the fish & pat it dry. Cut twelve 1- to 1 1/4-inch pieces. Place the fish in the bag. Seal by pressing out the air. Turn the fish gently to coat it in the marinade. Refrigerate for 30 to 1 hour. While the fish marinates, soak Twelve 6- to 8-inches wooden skewers in water.
3. Insert 2 pieces of pepper, 2 pieces of pineapple, and 1 piece of fish around each skewer in random order.

4. Make sure the grill is ready for direct cooking. Using nonstick frying spray, coat the grid. Place the grid 4–6 inches above the heat source. Heat the grill to medium-high. Arrange the skewers on the grid. Grill for around 3 to 4 minutes on medium-high heat, or until grill marks emerge on the bottom, covered or tenting with foil. Turn the skewers over and cook for another 3 to 4 minutes, or until the fish starts to flake when checked with a fork.

Scrumptious Tuna Cakes with Creamy Cucumber Dipping

Cooking time: 15 minutes

Preparation time: 10 minutes

Servings: 5

Per serving: Calories 187, Total fat 9g, Protein 13g, Carbs 13g

Ingredients:

- 1/3 cup of shredded carrots
- 1/2 cup of cucumber finely chopped
- 2 teaspoons of spicy brown mustard
- 1/2 cup of plain yogurt fat-free
- 1 tablespoon of olive oil or olive oil, divided
- 1 1/2 teaspoons of chopped fresh dill
- 1/4 cup of celery finely chopped
- Lemon wedges, optional
- 1/4 cup of sliced green onion
- 1 cup of panko bread crumbs, divided
- 1 teaspoon of lemon-pepper seasoning salt
- 1/4 cup of mayonnaise reduced-fat
- 1 can of albacore tuna in water 12 ounces, drained

Instructions:

Follow the instructions below to make a scrumptious tuna cake with creamy cucumber dipping.

1. To make the sauce, combine the cucumber, dill, yogurt, and lemon-pepper spice in a mixing bowl. Cover and chill until ready to serve.
2. Combine carrots, onion, mayonnaise, celery, and mustard in a mixing dish. 1/2 cup panko, stirred in. Mix in the tuna until everything is well mixed.

3. In a small-sized dish, place the remaining panko. Make 5 1/2-inch-thick patties out of the tuna mixture. Lightly coat the patties in panko.
4. Warm 1 1/2 teaspoons of oil in a 10-inch nonstick skillet Toss in the patties. Cook, uncovered, for 5 to 6 minutes on medium flame, or till golden brown, flipping once. When the patties are turned, add the rest of 1 1/2 teaspoon's oil to the skillet. Serve with the yogurt mixture and, if wanted, lemon slices.

Mouth-Watering Chicken Cutlets

Cooking time: 20 minutes

Preparation time: 10 minutes

Servings: 6

Per serving: Calories 269, Total fat 12g, Protein 28g, Carbs 14g

Ingredients:

- 1 cup of almond flour
- 1 tablespoon of garlic powder
- 1/2 teaspoon of ground black pepper
- 2 whole beaten eggs
- 1/2 teaspoon of Kosher salt
- 4 chicken breast boneless & skinless
- 2 tablespoons of olive oil

Instructions:

Follow the instructions below to make mouth-watering chicken cutlets.

1. Cut the chicken into tiny chunks using a sharp knife nugget-style
2. In a medium mixing dish, combine the garlic powder, almond flour, salt, and black pepper.
3. Dip the chicken chunks into the beaten eggs one at a time, then cover them in the flour mixture, shaking off any excess flour.
4. Coat the nonstick pan with two teaspoons of olive oil.
5. Add the chicken pieces & cook on a medium flame for around 20 minutes, or until golden brown.

Tasty Salmon Sandwiches with Apricot Sauce

Cooking time: 10 minutes

Preparation time: 10 minutes

Servings: 4

Per serving: Calories 269, Total fat 9g, Protein 24g, Carbs 23g

Ingredients:

- 1 small-sized lemon
- 4 lettuce leaves Nonstick cooking spray
- 2 tablespoons of sweet chili sauce
- Asian-style Aluminum foil
- 1/2 teaspoon of black pepper
- 1 pound of skinless Atlantic salmon,
- 4 square fillets 4 tablespoons of apricot preserve low-sugar
- 4 98% of fat-free light wheat sandwich buns

Instructions:

Follow the instructions below to make tasty salmon sandwiches with apricot sauce.

1. Preheat the grill, either indoors or outside. Spray a piece of aluminum foil big enough to contain the four fillets with nonstick cooking spray.
2. Place the fillets on foil & season with lemon juice & black pepper. Grill for 5 minutes on each side on foil until done through. Grill the buns or toast them in the toaster.
3. Top each of the base halves of the buns with a lettuce leaf, then one salmon fillet. Combine apricot preserves & sweet chili sauce in a small dish, then put about 1 heaping tablespoon upon each salmon fillet; top with the top 1/2 of each bun to finish.

Grilled Peaches Topped with Cream Cheese Spicy Topping

Cooking time: 10 minutes

Preparation time: 10 minutes

Servings: 6

Per serving: Calories 182, Total fat 6g, Protein 4g, Carbs 28g

Ingredients:

- 1/4 teaspoon ground red pepper
- 1/4 cup of toasted slivered almonds
- 1/2 cup of softened light cream cheese
- 4 ounces 6 peaches, halved & pits removed
- 1 tablespoon of stevia
- Fresh mint leaves optional
- 2 cups of thawed and frozen fat-free whipped topping

Instructions:

Follow the instructions below to make grilled peaches topped with cream cheese spicy topping.

1. On medium-high heat, prepare the grill for direct grilling. Using nonstick frying spray, coat the grid.
2. In a medium-sized mixing dish, gently whisk cream cheese until smooth. Blend in the stevia & ground red pepper till smooth. Lastly, fold in the whipped topping. Refrigerate till ready to use, covered.
3. Place the peaches on the grill, cut sides down. 2 to 3 minutes on the grill, covered. Turnover and cook for another 2 to 3 minutes, or until peaches soften. Transfer to a platter and set aside to cool slightly.
4. Place 2 peach halves on 6 plates, cut sides up. Spread the spicy cream cheese coating and almonds evenly on top. Garnish with a sprig of mint.

Tempting Salmon Croquettes

Cooking time: 20 minutes

Preparation time: 10 minutes

Servings: 9

Per serving: Calories 491, Total fat 34g, Protein 37g, Carbs 11g

Ingredients:

- 2 tablespoons of minced fresh chives
- 3 tablespoons of olive oil, divided
- 1 cup of panko bread crumbs
- 2 tablespoons of reduced-fat mayonnaise
- 2 teaspoons of lemon zest fresh
- 2 1/2 cups of flaked salmon or 175 ounces of can pink salmon, without bones
- 1 large beaten egg
- 1/4 teaspoon of black pepper
- 2 tablespoons of minced red bell pepper
- 1 tablespoon of lemon juice
- 1 clove of minced garlic
- 1 tablespoon of Dijon mustard
- 1 tablespoon of minced fresh parsley
- 1/4 teaspoon of kosher salt

Instructions:

Follow the instructions below to make tempting salmon croquettes.

1. Toss the egg, salmon, garlic, chives, panko bread crumbs, red bell pepper, reduced-fat mayonnaise, parsley, Dijon mustard, lemon juice, black pepper, lemon zest, kosher salt, and 1 tablespoon of olive oil together in a large-sized mixing dish.
2. Shape the mixture into 9 patties.

3. In a nonstick pan, warm two tablespoons of olive oil on medium flame and lay the patties in the pan. Cook for 15 minutes, then flip & cook for another 5 minutes, or until golden brown.

Tempting Mushroom Smothered Beef Patties

Cooking time: 25 minutes

Preparation time: 5 minutes

Servings: 4

Per serving: Calories 365, Total fat 23g, Protein 26g, Carbs 18g

Ingredients:

- 1 1/2 cups of mushrooms sliced
- 1 egg whisked
- 2 tablespoons of water
- 1 pound of ground beef
- 1 small onion chopped
- 3 tablespoon of olive oil, divided
- 1 tablespoon of Worcestershire sauce
- 1/3 cup of Italian-seasoned dry bread crumbs
- 1 can of Condensed Cream of Mushroom Soup Regular or 98% Fat-Free 75 ounces

Instructions:

Follow the instructions below to make tempting mushroom-smothered beef patties.

1. Combine the beef, crumbs, 1/4 cup of soup, egg, & onion in a large-sized dish. Make four patties out of the beef mixture.
2. Cook the patties in a skillet with two teaspoons of olive oil on a medium flame for around 15 minutes. Flip them on halfway through.
3. Heat 1 tablespoon of oil in a pan before adding the remaining soup & broth. Bring the mushrooms & Worcestershire sauce to a boil. Add the fried patties to the pan, covered them, & cook for 5 minutes on low flame.

Soy-Ginger Flavored Steak Bites

Cooking time: 20 minutes

Preparation time: 10 minutes

Servings: 6

Per serving: Calories 442, Total fat 30g, Protein 35g, Carbs 8g

Ingredients:

- 2 tablespoons of olive oil
- 1 1/2 pounds of sirloin steak/ribeye/strip loin
- 1 tablespoon of melted butter
- For the Marinade:
- 1 tablespoon of olive oil
- 2 tablespoons of stevia
- 1 teaspoon of fresh lemon juice
- 2 tablespoons of soy sauce
- 3 cloves of garlic minced
- 2 teaspoons of ginger fresh minced

Instructions:

Follow the instructions below to make soy-ginger flavored steak bites.

1. Before adding the steak bites, cut the steak into bite-size pieces and put all marinade ingredients in a mixing dish.
2. Chill for around 30 minutes to 2 hours in the refrigerator. Remove the steak bites from the marinade after 30 minutes.
3. In a skillet, warm 2 tablespoons of olive oil and add the steak bites. On medium flame, cook for 15 to 20 minutes. Finish with a drizzle of butter and sesame seeds, then serve and enjoy!

Steak, Chicken and Shrimp Skewers

Cooking time: 15 minutes

Preparation time: 15 minutes

Servings: 10 skewers

Per serving: Calories 222, Total fat 9g, Protein 26g, Carbs 8g

Ingredients:

- 20 large-sized shrimp
- 1/4 chopped yellow bell pepper
- 1 1/4 pounds of chicken thigh meat skinless, sliced into 20 one-ounce segments
- 3 chopped sweet chilies
- 1/2 cup of fresh cilantro leaves
- 11/4 pounds of lean skirt steak, fat removed, sliced into 10 two-ounce segments
- 1 green pepper
- 2 minced cloves of garlic
- 1 medium-sized papaya optional
- 1 chopped onion
- 1 red onion
- 1/4 chopped red bell pepper
- 1 tablespoon of vegetable oil
- 1/4 chopped green bell pepper

Instructions:

Follow the instructions below to make steak, chicken and shrimp skewers.

1. In a shallow dish, combine the steak pieces, chicken pieces, and shrimp pieces. In an electric blender, combine all of the sofrito ingredients. To make a coarse puree, combine all of the ingredients in a blender. Over the steak, chicken, and

shrimp, pour the entire contents of the blender. Refrigerate for 24 hours after covering & marinating.

2. Cut green pepper into 20 strips, red onion into 20 pieces, & papaya into 20 cubes when ready to grill skewers. To make the skewers, alternate two pieces of chicken, one steak, two shrimp, wedges of red onion, two strips of green pepper, two and two chunks of papaya onto each skewer for color and variety. Any remaining sofrito should be discarded. Arrange the skewers on a hot grill & cook for around 15 minutes, turning to keep the heat even, until the chicken & beef are cooked through. Alternatively, you can use the oven broiler to broil the skewers. Serve right away.

Mouth-Watering Beef Chimichangas

Cooking time: 10 minutes

Preparation time: 20 minutes

Servings: 6

Per serving: Calories 295, Total fat 12g, Protein 22g, Carbs 25g

Ingredients:

- 1 can of chopped green chilies 4 ounces
- 1/4 teaspoon of ground cumin
- 1 pound of lean ground beef 90% lean
- 3/4 cup of grated Monterey Jack cheese
- 1 chopped small onion
- Low-fat sour cream and guacamole, optional
- 2 minced garlic cloves
- 6 whole-wheat tortillas 8 inches
- 1/4 cup of salsa

Instructions:

Follow the instructions below to make mouth-watering beef chimichangas.

1. Cook the onion, beef, and garlic in a large-sized pan on a medium flame for 6 to 8 minutes, or until the beef is no pinker, and the onion is soft, breaking up the steak into crumbles; drain. Mix the salsa, chilies, and cumin.
2. Fill half cup of beef mixture in the middle of each tortilla; 2 tablespoons cheese on top. Fold the tortilla's bottom and edges over the filling and roll it up.
3. Place the chimichangas, seam side down, on the grill rack. Cover & grill for around 10 to 12 minutes on medium-low heat, flipping once, until crisp & brown. Serve them with sour cream & guacamole, if desired.

Appetizing Sirloin Steak Antipasto Salad

Cooking time: 15 minutes

Preparation time: 10 minutes

Servings: 4

Per serving: Calories 250, Total fat 7g, Protein 30g, Carbs 21g

Ingredients:
- 8 cups of torn romaine lettuce
- 3 minced cloves of garlic
- 1/3 cup Italian or Caesar salad dressing fat-free
- 16 pitted Kalamata olives, halved lengthwise
- 1/2 teaspoon of black pepper
- 1/4 cup of fresh basil, slice into thin strips
- 16 halved cherry tomatoes
- 1 beef top sirloin steak around 1 pound & 3/4-inch-thick, trimmed of fat
- 1 can of quartered artichoke hearts in water 14 ounces, rinsed & drained

Instructions:

Follow the instructions below to make an appetizing sirloin steak antipasto salad.

1. Preheat the broiler or prepare the grill for direct cooking. Season the meat with garlic & pepper.
2. Grill steaks on medium-hot coals for around 4 minutes on each side for medium-rare or till the desired doneness, or broil 4 inches from flame for 4 minutes per side. Place the steak on a chopping board and cover with foil. Allow for at least 5 minutes of resting time.
3. In a large-sized mixing bowl, combine the lettuce, olives, tomatoes, and artichoke hearts. Toss in the dressing. Place in four plates.
4. Cut steak into thin slices crosswise and serve over salads. Drizzle meat with juices from the cutting board. Garnish with basil leaves.

Cheddar and Asparagus Chicken Breasts

Cooking time: 25 minutes

Preparation time: 5 minutes

Servings: 4

Per serving: Calories 189, Total fat 4g, Protein 33g, Carbs 5g

Ingredients:

- 1 medium chopped red bell pepper
- 1/4 teaspoon of black pepper
- 20 asparagus spears around 2 bunches
- 4 tablespoons of corn relish optional
- 2 cups of fat-free and reduced-sodium chicken broth
- 4 tablespoons of grated low-fat Cheddar cheese
- 1 teaspoon of dried parsley
- 1/2 teaspoon of roasted and crushed garlic
- 4 boneless and skinless chicken breasts around 1/4 pound each

Instructions:

Follow the instructions below to make cheddar and asparagus chicken breasts.

1. Remove the woody stem ends from the asparagus and discard them. Set aside asparagus tips that are about 4 inches long. In a saucepan, combine asparagus stalks, broth, red pepper, parsley, garlic, and black pepper. Cook for 20 minutes at medium-high heat, stirring periodically.
2. Put each chicken breast half in plastic wrap and pound with a rolling pin until about 1/4-inch- thick while the vegetables simmer.
3. Preheat an indoor electric grill with a cover. 5 asparagus tips should be arranged on one end of the each pounded breast. Fold in half after adding 1 spoonful of cheese to each. Place

the stuffed breasts on the grill and cook for 6 minutes with the lid covered.
4. Place cooked breast on top of veggie sauce on serving dishes. If desired, top with corn relish.

Tasty Polenta Triangles

Cooking time: 25 minutes

Preparation time: 5 minutes

Servings: 8

Per serving: Calories 62, Total fat 2g, Protein 3g, Carbs 9g

Ingredients:
- 1/2 cup of crumbled feta cheese 2 ounces
- 1/2 cup of yellow corn grits uncooked
- 2 cloves of minced garlic
- 1 1/2 cups fat-free reduced-sodium chicken broth, divided
- 1 peeled & finely chopped red bell pepper, roasted

Instructions:

Follow the instructions below to make tasty polenta triangles.

1. In a small-sized mixing bowl, combine grits & 1/2 cup of chicken broth; stir well. Bring the leftover 1 cup broth to a boil in a big heavy pot. Mix in the garlic & wet grits thoroughly. Bring the water back to a boil. Reduce the flame to a low setting. Cook for 15 minutes with the lid on. Remove from heat and stir in the feta cheese. Stir until all of the cheese has melted. Mix in the roasted bell pepper well.
2. Using nonstick cooking spray, coat an 8-inch square baking pan. Pour the grit mixture into the pan that has been prepared. Push grits uniformly into the pan with damp fingertips. Refrigerate until completely chilled.
3. Using nonstick frying spray, coat the grid. Make sure the grill is ready for direct cooking. Cut polenta into 2-inch squares after turning it out onto a cutting board. Each square should be cut diagonally into two triangles.
4. Arrange the polenta triangles on the grid. Grill for 1 minute over medium-high heat or until the bottoms are gently

browned. Grill the triangles on the other side till browned and crisp.

Oatmeal and Apple Cookie Crumble

Cooking time: 18 minutes

Preparation time: 10 minutes

Servings: 6

Per serving: Calories 169, Total fat 5g, Protein 4g, Carbs 32g

Ingredients:

- 1/2 teaspoon of ground cinnamon
- 6 cups of diced and unpeeled apples
- 3/4 cup of oatmeal cookie mix
- 1/4 cup of water
- 1 tablespoon of olive oil
- 1/3 cup of raisins
- 1 teaspoon of vanilla, nut and butter flavoring or 1 1/2 teaspoons of vanilla

Instructions:

Follow the instructions below to make oatmeal and apple cookie crumble.

1. At 400°F, preheat the oven. Using nonstick cooking spray, coat a 117-inch baking pan. In a large-sized mixing dish, combine the apples, water, cinnamon, raisins, and flavoring. Place in a pan. Set the pan aside.
2. In a medium-sized mixing dish, stir together the cookie mix & oil with a fork until thoroughly combined. Over the apple mixture, sprinkle evenly. Bake for around 17 minutes, or till apples are soft. Allow 30 minutes to rest before serving.

Tempting Caprese Portobello Burgers

Cooking time: 15 minutes

Preparation time: 10 minutes

Servings: 4

Per serving: Calories 198, Total fat 6g, Protein 13g, Carbs 28g

Ingredients:

- 2 chopped plum tomatoes
- 1/8 teaspoon of black pepper
- 4 Portobello mushrooms around
- 3/4 pound, gills & stems removed
- 1 tablespoon of light balsamic vinaigrette
- 3 ounces of diced mozzarella cheese
- 4 toasted whole wheat sandwich thin rounds
- 1 clove of crushed garlic
- 2 tablespoons of chopped fresh basil

Instructions:

Follow the instructions below to make tempting Caprese Portobello burgers.

1. Coat the grill with cooking spray & heat it to medium-high. In a small bowl, combine the cheese, tomatoes, garlic, basil, vinaigrette, and pepper.
2. Grill mushroom caps for Five minutes on each side, stem side down, or until done. Fill each cap with one-fourth of the tomato mixture. Cover and cook for 3 minutes, or until the cheese melts. Serve on a bed of thinly sliced bread.

Toothsome Crispy Chicken Bites

Cooking time: 15 minutes

Preparation time: 10 minutes

Servings: 8

Per serving: Calories 255, Total fat 2g, Protein 33g, Carbs 17g

Ingredients:
- 2 whole beaten eggs
- 1/2 teaspoon of Kosher salt
- 3/4 cup of almond flour
- 1 teaspoon of paprika
- 1/2 teaspoon of black pepper
- 1/2 teaspoon of dried rosemary
- 2 lbs. of chicken, sliced into small pieces
- 3/4 cup of breadcrumbs
- 1/2 teaspoon of dried thyme
- 2 tablespoons of olive oil

Instructions:

Follow the instructions below to make toothsome crispy chicken bites.

1. Sprinkle the all-purpose flour with salt and black pepper in a medium-sized mixing bowl.
2. Divide the eggs & breadcrumbs evenly among two serving dishes. In the beaten eggs dish, combine the paprika and spices.
3. Coat the chicken tenders in seasoned flour before dipping them in the egg mixture & rolling them in breadcrumbs.
4. In a nonstick skillet, warm two tablespoons of olive oil and cook the chicken tenders for 10 to 12 minutes, or till golden brown on both sides, rotating halfway through.

Mediterranean-Style Turkey Burgers with Feta

Cooking time: 15 minutes

Preparation time: 10 minutes

Servings: 4

Per serving: Calories 292, Total fat 10g, Protein 30g, Carbs 21g

Ingredients:

- 1/4 cup of red onion diced
- 1/4 cup of chopped and pitted Kalamata olives
- 4 white turkey burgers 95% lean
- 1/4 cup chopped cucumber
- 1/3 cup of plain non-fat yogurt
- 26-inch whole-wheat pita bread rounds, halved & warmed
- 1/4 cup of plum tomato diced
- 1/4 cup of fat-free feta cheese crumbled

Instructions:

Follow the instructions below to make Mediterranean-style turkey burgers with feta.

1. Grill burgers for 6 to 8 minutes per side on medium heat, or until completely cooked 165°F, rotating twice.
2. In a small-sized bowl, combine the yogurt, onion, tomato, olives, cucumber, and feta. In pita halves, serve the burgers and feta mixture.

Beef, Lamb and Pork Recipes

Tempting Beef Sirloin with a Green Salad

Cooking time: 25 minutes

Preparation time: 5 minutes

Servings: 4

Per serving: Calories 726, Total fat 45g, Protein 75g, Carbs 6g

Ingredients:
- 2 tablespoons of olive oil
- 1.5 kg sirloin of beef Small rocket bag
- Salt & freshly ground pepper
- For the green salad:
- 4 finely chopped spring onions
- Juice of a lemon
- 5 tablespoons of finely chopped capers
- 3 tablespoons of finely chopped gherkins
- 5 tablespoons of extra-virgin olive oil
- 1 tablespoon of finely chopped parsley

Instructions:

Follow the instructions below to make tempting beef sirloin with a green salad.

1. At 450°F, preheat the oven.
2. Rub the meat with the oil.
3. Then add salt and black pepper to taste.
4. Cook for 10 minutes in the oven with the meat on a baking pan. Reduce the oven temperature to 400°F and roast for 15 minutes. Remove from the oven and set aside to cool.
5. For the green salad: In a mixing dish, combine the capers, gherkins, spring onions, lemon juice, freshly cut parsley, and extra virgin olive oil.
6. Place the steak on a platter and slice it into thin slithers.
7. Top with a dollop of salsa Verde and a sprinkling of rocket leaves.

Delicious Lamb Curry

Cooking time: 25 minutes

Preparation time: 5 minutes

Servings: 2

Per serving: Calories 506, Total fat 36g, Protein 36g, Carbs 16g

Ingredients:

- 2 carrots, chopped into
- 1/2-inch slices
- 2 teaspoons of ground cumin
- 5 tablespoons of finely chopped parsley
- 2 tablespoons of olive oil
- 1 large finely chopped tomato
- 300 g of cubed lean lamb
- Salt & freshly ground black pepper to taste
- 1 finely chopped onion
- 1/2 teaspoon of turmeric
- 4 finely chopped garlic cloves
- 1/2 teaspoon of ground coriander
- 500 ml of hot chicken stock

Instructions:

Follow the instructions below to make delicious lamb curry.

1. In a large-sized saucepan, heat the oil at medium-high flame.
2. Add the lamb & brown all over when it's heated. This should take no more than 5 minutes. Sauté for around 3 minutes after adding the onion and finely chopped garlic.
3. The carrots, ground cumin, heated chicken stock, turmeric, and ground coriander should all be added at this point.
4. Bring everything to a boil.

5. Reduce the flame to low, cover, and cook for 15 minutes. Cook for 2 minutes after adding the chopped tomato & parsley. To taste, sprinkle with salt and pepper.

Sage and Lemon Pork

Cooking time: 25 minutes

Preparation time: 5 minutes

Servings: 4

Per serving: Calories 442, Total fat 12g, Protein 45g, Carbs 30.8g

Ingredients:

- 2 teaspoons of dried sage
- 2 x 200 g of pork tenderloin
- 250 g of carrots
- 200 g of Mascarpone cheese
- 300 g of celeriac
- Rind & juice of a lemon
- 250 g of peas
- 200 g of Parma Ham

Instructions:

Follow the instructions below to make sage and lemon pork. At 400°F, preheat the oven.

1. Using a sharp knife, cut the pork tenderloin in 1/2 lengthwise.
2. In a dish, combine the lemon rind, mascarpone, lemon juice, and sage. Fill the pork incision with the cheese mixture.
3. Wrap the pork in Parma ham and bake for around 25 minutes in a roasting tray in a preheated oven.
4. Cover the carrots, celeriac, and peas with water for the vegetables. Bring a pot of water to a boil.
5. Then reduce the flame to low and simmer the vegetables for 5 minutes. Slice the pork and serve with delicious vegetables!

Tasty Beef Teriyaki

Cooking time: 25 minutes

Preparation time: 5 minutes

Servings: 4

Per serving: Calories 478, Total fat 22g, Protein 38g, Carbs 26g

Ingredients:

- 1 salad onion
- 2 tablespoons of toasted sesame seeds, toasted
- 500 g of beef rump steak

FOR THE TERIYAKI SAUCE:

- 4 teaspoons of toasted sesame oil
- 120 ml of soy sauce
- 2 tablespoons of agave nectar
- 4 minced garlic cloves
- 4 tablespoons of rice mirin
- 1 tablespoon of clear honey

Instructions:

Follow the instructions below to make tasty beef teriyaki.

1. Combine the soy sauce, rice mirin, sesame oil, agave nectar, honey, and garlic cloves in a large-sized mixing dish.
2. Cut the beef & spring onions and mix with the sauce. Put in the fridge for around one hour, covered with cling film.
3. Remove the mixture and lay it on a griddle pan to cook for around 5 minutes, or until thoroughly done.
4. Spread the teriyaki sauce on top, sprinkle with sesame seeds, and enjoy!

Prosciutto and Tomato Panini Sandwiches

Cooking time: 15 minutes

Preparation time: 5 minutes

Servings: 4

Per serving: Calories 230, Total fat 8g, Protein 21g, Carbs 25g

Ingredients:

- 3 ounces of prosciutto thinly sliced
- 12 ounces of multigrain Italian bread
- 1 ounce of fresh baby spinach
- 1/2 teaspoon of chopped fresh rosemary
- 1/4 cup 2 ounces of grated reduced-fat mozzarella cheese
- 1/2 cup of chopped fresh basil leaves
- 1/4 cup of balsamic vinegar
- 2 medium tomatoes, thinly sliced 8 ounces in total

Instructions:

Follow the instructions below to make prosciutto and tomato panini sandwiches.

1. Bread should be cut in half lengthwise. Leave a 1/2-inch-thick shell after hollowing out the top and bottom portions. Save the broken bread for another occasion. Cover the bottom of the bread with cheese.
2. Toss the spinach with the balsamic vinegar. Tomatoes, prosciutto, rosemary, basil, and spinach are uniformly distributed on the bread. Cover with the remaining half of the bread. Cut the filled bread into four equal pieces crosswise.
3. Heat a grill pan on medium heat with nonstick cooking spray. Place the sandwiches in the pan. Place a cast-iron skillet or another heavy skillet over the sandwiches and

gently push to flatten them. Cook for 3 minutes, then flip and cook for another 2 minutes, or until the bread is toasted.

Flavorsome Spicy Beef Stew

Cooking time: 25 minutes

Preparation time: 5 minutes

Servings: 4

Per serving: Calories 338, Total fat 14g, Protein 33g, Carbs 21g

Ingredients:

- 1 finely chopped green chili
- 2 tablespoons of olive oil
- 400 g of tinned tomatoes
- 1 finely chopped medium onion
- 1 tablespoon of fresh coriander
- 3 finely chopped garlic cloves
- 1 sliced celery stick
- Salt & freshly ground pepper to taste
- 2 medium sliced red bell peppers
- 500 g of lean beef mince
- 400 g of cannellini beans

Instructions:

Follow the instructions below to make flavorsome spicy beef stew.

1. In a large-sized saucepan on medium heat, heat the vegetable oil & cook the onions for around 2 minutes.
2. Cook for another 2 minutes after adding the garlic & chili. Cook for 4 minutes after adding the red bell peppers & celery.
3. In a large-sized skillet, brown the lean beef mince on all sides. It takes roughly 4-5 minutes to do this task.
4. After that, add the tomatoes & beans. Reduce the flame to low and cook for around 20 minutes. Serve with brown basmati rice and salsa on the side.

Pork and Plum Kebabs

Cooking time: 15 minutes

Preparation time: 15 minutes

Servings: 4 2 kebabs: Calories 191, Total fat 5g, Protein 19g, Carbs 17g

Ingredients:

- 1 1/2 teaspoons of ground cumin
- 1/4 cup of green onions sliced
- 3/4 pound of pork loin chops boneless 1-inch-thick, trimmed & slice into1-inch pieces
- 1 tablespoon of orange juice
- 1/2 teaspoon of ground cinnamon
- 1/4 teaspoon of garlic powder
- 1/4 cup of raspberry fruit spread
- 1/4 teaspoon of salt
- 3 plums or nectarines, pitted & cut into wedges
- 1/4 teaspoon of ground red pepper

Instructions:

Follow the instructions below to make pork and plum kebabs.

1. Fill a big resealable bag halfway with meat. In a small-sized bowl, combine cumin, garlic powder, cinnamon, salt, and red pepper; pour over pork. Close the bag and shake it to coat the meat in spices.
2. In a small-sized bowl, combine fruit spread, green onions, and orange juice; leave aside.
3. Make sure the grill is ready for direct cooking. Attach pork & plum wedges alternately onto eight skewers. Grill kabobs for 12 to 14 minutes on medium heat, rotating once, or till meat is cooked through. During the last 5 minutes of cooking, brush the raspberry mixture on regularly.

Pork Chops Grilled with Cherry Sauce

Cooking time: 20 minutes

Preparation time: 10 minutes

Servings: 4

Per serving: Calories 187, Total fat 3g, Protein 29g, Carbs 11g

Ingredients:

- 4 ounces of apple juice unsweetened
- 1 tablespoon of honey
- 12 stemmed & pitted cherries
- 1 tablespoon of cornstarch
- 1–1 1/4 pounds of boneless lean pork chops
- 1 teaspoon of balsamic vinegar
- 1/4 teaspoon of thyme

Instructions:

Follow the instructions below to make pork chops grilled with cherry sauce.

1. In a small-sized saucepan on low flame, combine cherries & apple juice and cook for 15 minutes.
2. Preheat the grill while you're cooking the sauce. Grill chops for around 3 to 4 minutes on each side on the grill until pork chops are done through internal temperature ought to be 160°F.
3. Add the thyme, balsamic vinegar, honey, and cornstarch to the hot apple juice and cherries in a small food processor. Pulse just a few times. Return the sauce to the pot and cook, constantly stirring, for 3 minutes, or until it has thickened.
4. Serve cooked pork chops with sauce about 1/2 cup.

Jalapenos Beef Cheeseburgers

Cooking time: 10 minutes

Preparation time: 5 minutes

Servings: 4

Per serving: Calories 365, Total fat 21g, Protein 28g, Carbs 16g

Ingredients:

- 1 pound of 85% lean ground beef
- 4 tomato slices
- 4 drops of liquid hot pepper sauce
- 2 ounces 4 slices of Sargento Deli-Style low-fat
- Pepper Jack Cheese
- 1/4 cup of cilantro lightly chopped
- 4 whole-grain, light hamburger buns

Instructions:

Follow the instructions below to make jalapenos beef cheeseburgers.

1. Preheat the grill to high. Using a half-inch cutter, slice cheese into half-inch pieces. Combine the ground beef, cheese, and spicy pepper sauce in a medium-sized mixing dish and stir well.
2. Make four equal patties out of the meat. Depress the middle of each patty slightly.
3. Grill the burgers for about 5 minutes on each side, or until the meat is well cooked. Place the burger on the bottom of the hamburger bun and top with 1 tomato slice & a quarter of the cilantro.
4. Serve with the top bun.

Beef Stuffed Eggplants

Cooking time: 25 minutes

Preparation time: 5 minutes

Servings: 4

Per serving: Calories 195, Total fat 5g, Protein 25g, Carbs 12g

Ingredients:
- 2 halved lengthwise eggplants around 8 to 12 ounces each
- 1 teaspoon of black pepper
- 1/4 cup of water
- Nonstick cooking spray
- 2 cups of sliced green and red bell peppers
- 1 teaspoon of salt
- Chopped fresh parsley
- 1 1/2 teaspoons of chopped garlic
- 1 pound of boneless beef sirloin steak, trimmed of visible fat & cut into1/4-inch strips
- 2 cups of sliced mushrooms
- Pinch of paprika

Instructions:

Follow the instructions below to make beef stuffed eggplants.

1. At 450°F, preheat the oven. Coat a baking dish with nonstick cooking spray.
2. In a large-sized baking dish, place the eggplant halves face-up. In about 8 places, pierce the sliced sides with a fork. Sprinkle 1/4 teaspoon salt on each half of the eggplant. Bake for 10 minutes, covered with foil.
3. Spray a big nonstick skillet using cooking spray in the meantime. Cook, occasionally stirring, for 2 minutes over medium heat with the garlic & black pepper. Cook and stir for 5 minutes after adding the beef.

4. Cook for 5 minutes after adding the bell peppers. Cook for 5 minutes after adding the mushrooms. Stir in the water and cover. Turn off the flame in the skillet.
5. Take eggplant from the oven and set aside for 5 minutes to cool. Cooked eggplant centers should be mashed with a fork, but the shells should not be broken.
6. Top one-fourth of the beef mixture on each side; combine with mashed eggplant. Bake for 5 minutes after covering with foil. Remove the dish from the oven. Paprika and parsley are optional garnishes.

Marinated Mini Beef Skewers

Cooking time: 15 minutes

Preparation time: 15 minutes

Servings: 6

Per serving: Calories 120, Total fat 4g, Protein 20g, Carbs 2g

Ingredients:

- 1 teaspoon of dark sesame oil
- 1 beef top round steak around 1 pound
- 18 cherry tomatoes
- 2 tablespoons of low-sodium soy sauce
- 2 minced cloves of garlic
- 1 tablespoon of dry sherry

Instructions:

Follow the instructions below to make marinated mini beef skewers.

1. 18 1/8-inch-thick slices of beef, cut crosswise and fill a big resealable with beef. In a small- sized cup, combine the soy sauce, oil, sherry, and garlic; pour over the beef. Close the bag and turn it over to coat. Refrigerate for at least 30 minutes, but up to 2 hours.
2. Meanwhile, soak 18 wooden skewers 6 inches in water for 20 minutes.
3. Preheat the oven to broil. Drain the beef & toss out the marinade. Accordion-style weave the steak onto the skewers. Place on broiler pan's rack.
4. Broil for 2 minutes at 4 to 5 inches from the heat source. Turn the skewers over and broil for another 2 minutes, or until the beef is slightly pink.
5. One cherry tomato should be placed on each skewer. Warm the dish before serving.

Balsamic Beef, Onion and Mushrooms

Cooking time: 25 minutes

Preparation time: 5 minutes

Servings: 4

Per serving: Calories 216, Total fat 9g, Protein 26g, Carbs 7g

Ingredients:

- 4 to 5 teaspoons of balsamic vinegar, divided
- 2 large sliced sweet onions
- 1/4 teaspoon of dried thyme
- 3 teaspoons of olive oil, divided
- 1 boneless beef top sirloin around 1 pound, slice into 1/2-inch-thick slices
- 1/4 to 1/2 teaspoon of black pepper
- 1/2 teaspoon of salt, divided
- 3 ounces around 1 cup of sliced mushrooms

Instructions:

Follow the instructions below to make balsamic beef, onion and mushrooms.

1. On medium flame, heat a large-sized nonstick skillet. Cook and stir for 15 minutes after adding the onions.
2. Put in 2 teaspoons of oil & 1/4 teaspoon of salt, stirred together 3 teaspoons of balsamic vinegar, one teaspoon at a time, scraping out browned pieces with a spatula.
3. Reduce the flame to a medium-low setting. Cook, occasionally stirring, for 4 to 5 minutes, or till mushrooms are soft. Place in a medium mixing dish. Set aside, covered.
4. Raise the temperature to medium-high. Mix 1 teaspoon of leftover oil. Sprinkle the remaining 1/4 teaspoon salt, thyme, and black pepper over the beef. Cook for 4–6 minutes, or until golden brown.

5. Turn the flame off. Over the steak, drizzle the remaining 2 teaspoons of balsamic vinegar. Toss in the veggies. Serve right away.

Appetizing Lamb Shashlik

Cooking time: 15 minutes

Preparation time: 10 minutes

Servings: 4

Per serving: Calories 250, Total fat 12g, Protein 22g, Carbs 4g

Ingredients:

- 3 sprigs of rosemary
- 500 g of diced lamb
- 1 lemon juice
- Salt & freshly ground pepper to taste
- 2 onions, sliced into wedges
- 8 BBQ skewers
- 1 yellow, 1 red, and 1 green bell pepper, diced
- 4 teaspoons of finely chopped garlic
- 3 tablespoons of olive oil

Instructions:

Follow the instructions below to make appetizing lamb shashlik.

1. Combine the lamb, lemon juice, oil, garlic, and rosemary in a large-sized mixing dish. Refrigerate for a couple of hours after covering.
2. Thread a piece of lamb, a slice of red bell pepper, a piece of onion, and a slice of green pepper onto your BBQ skewers.
3. Rep till the skewer is completely packed.
4. Arrange the lamb on the grill and cook for 5 minutes, or until the color changes. Then flip it overcook for another 5-10 minutes, or until done to your liking.
5. Insert a skewer or knife into the lamb to see if it is fully done.
6. If the juice is bloody, the meat isn't fully done. If the fluid is clear, though, the lamb is cooked.

Balsamic Pork Chops Grilled

Cooking time: 15 minutes

Preparation time: 10 minutes

Servings: 2

Per serving: Calories 196, Total fat 5g, Protein 26g, Carbs 8g

Ingredients:

- 2 tablespoons of low-sodium soy sauce
- 1/8 teaspoon of red pepper flakes
- 2 tablespoons of balsamic vinegar
- 2 pork chops boneless, trimmed of fat around 8 ounces in total
- 2 teaspoons of stevia
- 1 teaspoon of Dijon mustard

Instructions:

Follow the instructions below to make balsamic pork chops grilled.

1. In a small-sized dish, combine the vinegar, stevia, soy sauce, mustard, and red pepper flakes. Stir until everything is completely combined. 1 tablespoon marinade should be kept in the fridge until used.
2. Fill a big resealable bag halfway with meat. Pour the remaining sauce over the pork. Close the bag and turn it over to coat. Refrigerate for at least 2 hours or overnight.
3. Heat a grill pan on a medium-high flame, sprayed with nonstick cooking spray. Remove the pork from the marinade & discard it. Cook for around 4 minutes on each side, or until the middle is just slightly pink. Place on plates and drizzle with the remaining 1 tablespoon marinade.

Garlic Beef Brochettes Grilled

Cooking time: 15 minutes

Preparation time: 10 minutes

Servings: 4

Per serving: Calories 252, Total fat 12g, Protein 27g, Carbs 8g

Ingredients:

- 3 cloves of minced garlic
- 1 small-sized red onion, slice into 1/2-inch-thick wedges
- 2 tablespoons of chopped fresh thyme
- 1/3 cup of light Caesar salad dressing
- 1 large yellow or red bell pepper or 1/2 of each, slice into 1-inch chunks
- 1 pound of beef tenderloin tips or steaks, slice into 1 1/2-inch pieces

Instructions:

Follow the instructions below to make garlic beef brochettes grilled.

1. Preheat the grill to medium-high. In a small-sized bowl, combine the dressing & garlic. Mix in the onion, tenderloin, and bell pepper; toss well to coat, then set aside for 20 minutes.
2. Attach meat and veggies alternately onto four long metal skewers. Any leftover marinade from the meal should be brushed over the meat and veggies.
3. Grill skewers for Five minutes on each side on a covered grill. The tenderloin should be pink in the middle and the veggies crisp-tender. Finish with a sprig of thyme.

Tempting Lamb Kebabs with Verdant Salsa

Cooking time: 15 minutes

Preparation time: 10 minutes

Servings: 4

Per serving: Calories 300, Total fat 21g, Protein 18g, Carbs 9g

Ingredients:

For the kebabs:

- 1 tablespoon of finely chopped fresh coriander
- 2 teaspoons of peeled & finely chopped garlic
- 1/4 teaspoon of ground black pepper
- 1 peeled and finely chopped large onion
- 2 teaspoons of ground cumin
- 400 g of minced lamb
- 4 metal skewers
- 2 teaspoons of peeled & finely chopped ginger
- 2 teaspoons of ground coriander

For the verdant salsa:

- 1 bunch of chopped parsley
- 3 chopped spring onions
- 1 tablespoon of pitted olives of your choice
- 1 tablespoon of olive oil
- Juice & grated rind of a lemon
- 4 roughly chopped tomatoes
- 1 bunch of chopped coriander

Instructions:

Follow the instructions below to make tempting lamb kebabs with verdant salsa.

1. In a mixing dish, combine the mince, onion, ginger, garlic, pepper, coriander, cumin, and salt. Form the mince mixture into 16 balls.
2. Flatten each ball by wrapping it around the point of a metal skewer.
3. Refrigerate the meatballs for an hour after placing them on a baking sheet & covering them. Combine all of the salsa ingredients in a mixing dish.
4. Grill the skewered lamb kebabs underneath a hot grill, occasionally flipping until the meat is thoroughly cooked.
5. It will take around 15 minutes to complete this task. Serve immediately with salsa.

Caramelized Onion and Brie Burgers

Cooking time: 20 minutes

Preparation time: 10 minutes

Servings: 6

Per serving: Calories 432, Total fat 25g, Protein 42g, Carbs 5g

Ingredients:

For the onions:

- 1/2 teaspoon of salt
- 2 tablespoons of olive oil
- 1 thinly sliced large onion

For the mushrooms:

- 226 g of sliced mushrooms
- 2 tablespoons of butter

For the burgers:

- 125 g of brie cheese, sliced into small pieces
- 1/2 teaspoon of salt
- 900 g of ground beef
- 1/2 teaspoon of ground pepper

Instructions:

Follow the instructions below to make caramelized onion and brie burgers.

1. Preheat the grill to medium-high temperature.
2. In a large-sized frying pan, warm the olive oil and sauté the onions with a touch of salt for 5 minutes, or until soft and caramel brown in the shade. Don't allow them to become crispy!
3. Remove the onions to a platter & keep the pan available for frying the mushrooms.

4. In a large-sized mixing bowl, combine the beef, salt, and black pepper for the burgers. Hand-mix to thoroughly combine, then split into 6 equal halves.
5. Make a thin patty out of half of each component.
6. To make your burger, the top half of each thin patty with brie & onions, and top with the other half, laying the 2nd patty on top of the cheese & onions.
7. Cook the burgers for 4-5 minutes on each side on a hot grill.
8. Sauté the mushrooms in the little butter for 2-3 minutes while the burgers grilling. Remove the burgers from the grill once they've finished cooking.
9. Serve with a side salad and mushrooms and onions on top of the grilled burgers.

Tasty Lamb Meatballs

Cooking time: 20 minutes

Preparation time: 10 minutes

Servings: 5

Per serving: Calories 216, Total fat 15g, Protein 19g, Carbs 6g

Ingredients:

- 3 teaspoons of finely chopped garlic
- 2 green chilies
- 1/4 teaspoon of ground black pepper
- 400 g of minced lamb
- 3 teaspoons of ground coriander
- 2 finely chopped small onions
- 8 BBQ skewers
- 3 teaspoons of finely chopped ginger
- Salt to season
- 3 teaspoons of ground cumin
- 1 tablespoon of finely chopped fresh coriander

Instructions:

Follow the instructions below to make tasty lamb meatballs.

1. In a large-sized mixing bowl, thoroughly combine the mince, garlic, onion, ginger, chilies, ground cumin, salt, ground coriander, fresh coriander, and pepper.
2. Refrigerate this mixture for at least an hour.
3. After an hour, remove the mix from the fridge & roll it into 16 balls.
4. Form each ball into a four-inch or 10 cm long oval by wrapping it around the point of a metal skewer.
5. Grill the skewered meatballs over a hot grill or on a hot barbeque. Turn the meatballs frequently until they are fully cooked.

6. This will take about 15 minutes.
7. Savour with a dollop of handmade tomato ketchup.

No-Cook Sweet and Sour Ham Kebabs

Cooking time: 0 minutes

Preparation time: 10 minutes

Servings: 2 kebabs

Per serving: Calories 233, Total fat 9g, Protein 16g, Carbs 22g

Ingredients:

- 6 cherry tomatoes
- 4 1-inch ham chunks 1/2 ounce each
- 2 tablespoons of sweet 'n sour dressing
- 1/3 green bell pepper, sliced into four strips
- 2 ten-inch skewers
- 4 1-inch pineapple chunks around 1/4 cup

Instructions:

Follow the instructions below to make no-cook sweet and sour ham kebabs.

1. Arrange a tomato, a pepper strip, a pineapple chunk, and a ham cube on each skewer. Rep with a tomato at the end. Drizzle the dressing over the kabobs in a shallow dish. If desired, cover and chill for 1-2 hours to allow the flavors to meld.

Lamb Steak with a Tomato Sauce

Cooking time: 20 minutes

Preparation time: 10 minutes

Servings: 4

Per serving: Calories 198, Total fat 6g, Protein 23g, Carbs 5g

Ingredients:

- 400 g tin of chopped tomatoes
- Salt & freshly ground pepper to taste
- 1 finely chopped clove of garlic
- 4 lamb leg steaks
- A sprig of fresh coriander for garnish
- 1 teaspoon of cumin seeds
- 2 tablespoons of olive oil
- 1 teaspoon of ground coriander

Instructions:

Follow the instructions below to make lamb steak with a tomato sauce.

2. Cook the lamb steaks in a medium-sized pan with a tablespoon of oil until brown on both sides, about 5 minutes.
3. Spread the lamb steaks on kitchen paper to drain after they've been cooked. In a medium-sized pan, heat the remaining tablespoon of oil.
4. For about a minute, fry the seasonings.
5. Combine the chopped tomatoes with the spices in the pan and stir well. The dish should then be simmered for 10 minutes on low flame.
6. Add some water if the stew thickens until the lamb is fully cooked. Serve with a side of salad & freshly chopped coriander.

Fish And Seafood Recipes

COD with Spinach and Garlic

Cooking time: 25 minutes

Preparation time: 5 minutes

Servings: 4

Per serving: Calories 340, Total fat 16g, Protein 49g, Carbs 6g

Ingredients:

- 3 crushed garlic cloves
- Salt & freshly ground pepper
- 720 g of fresh baby leaf spinach, rinsed
- 200 g of vine tomatoes
- 3 tablespoons of olive oil
- 4 cod fillets around 180g each

Instructions:

Follow the instructions below to make COD with spinach and garlic.

1. At 450°F, preheat the oven.
2. In a frying pan on medium flame, add 2 tablespoons of oil. Add the crushed garlic cloves & the rinsed spinach.
3. To wilt the spinach, cook for 5 minutes. Once this is done, lightly grease a baking tray.
4. Drizzle the tomatoes with olive oil and place them on the baking tray. The cooking time is 10 minutes.
5. For the last 15 minutes, add the cod & tomatoes, seasoning with salt and freshly ground black pepper.
6. Serve the fish with the tomatoes on a bed of wilted spinach.

Tasty Chili Prawns

Cooking time: 10 minutes

Preparation time: 10 minutes

Servings: 4

Per serving: Calories 162, Total fat 13g, Protein 15g, Carbs 2g

Ingredients:

- 3 tablespoons of olive oil
- 1 lemon juice
- 300 g of tiger or king prawns cooked
- 2 tablespoons of sweet chili sauce
- 8 BBQ skewers
- 1 tablespoon of Dijon mustard

Instructions:

Follow the instructions below to make tasty chili prawns.

1. To make a marinade for the prawns, whisk together the olive oil, lemon juice, Dijon mustard, & sweet chili sauce in a mixing dish.
2. Add the prawns once the marinade has reached an even texture & color. Toss the prawns in the sauce until they're completely covered.
3. Set aside for approximately an hour in the refrigerator. Overnight is the best option. String the marinated prawns onto skewers and set them on a flat platter to grill.
4. Grill the skewered prawns for a total of 5 minutes, or until they start to caramelize on the outside.

Trout Fish with Beans

Cooking time: 10 minutes

Preparation time: 10 minutes

Servings: 4

Per serving: Calories 703, Total fat 36g, Protein 61g, Carbs 32g

Ingredients:

- 4 tablespoons of extra virgin olive oil
- Juice of 1 lemon
- 400 g of tinned cannellini beans, drained
- Salt & freshly ground pepper to taste
- 4 x 250 g of trout fillets
- 2 fresh green chilies, deseeded & finely chopped
- 400 g of tinned kidney beans, drained
- A handful of finely chopped fresh mint
- 1 tablespoon of finely chopped garlic cloves

Instructions:

Follow the instructions below to make trout fish with beans. At 360°F, preheat the oven.

1. In a mixing dish, combine the green chilies, drained cannellini beans, and mint. Using a tablespoon of olive oil, lightly sprinkle the fish fillets.
2. Season the fish with salt and black pepper after sprinkling the garlic on top. Bake the fillets for 10 minutes in a preheated oven.
3. Remove from the oven and drizzle with a tablespoon of extra virgin olive oil & lemon juice. To taste, season with salt & pepper.
4. Enjoy on top of a bed of beans!

Roasted Whole Lemon Sole with Celeriac

Cooking time: 25 minutes

Preparation time: 5 minutes

Servings: 4

Per serving: Calories 450, Total fat 29g, Protein 22g, Carbs 24g

Ingredients:

- 350 g of cherry tomatoes
- Zest & juice of 1 lemon
- 8x 260 g of lemon sole
- 12 fresh thyme leaves
- 800 g of celeriac
- Salt & freshly ground black pepper
- 8 tablespoons of olive oil

Instructions:

Follow the instructions below to make a roasted whole lemon sole with celeriac.

1. At 360°F, preheat the oven.
2. Celeriac should be peeled and diced into small bits.
3. Drizzle a tablespoon of olive oil over the cherry tomatoes on a baking sheet. Around 15 minutes, roast them.
4. Remove them from the oven and set them aside to cool.
5. In a large-sized frying pan on medium flame, heat a tablespoon of olive oil, then fried the lemon soles one at a time in the oil. The Lemon sole should be fried for about 5 minutes on each side.
6. When they're all done, serve them and season to taste with salt and black pepper. With roasted celeriac & orange tomatoes, serve the fillets.

BBQ Shrimps with Tropical Rice

Cooking time: 15 minutes

Preparation time: 10 minutes

Servings: 4

Per serving: Calories 200, Total fat 2g, Protein 9g, Carbs 37g

Ingredients:

- 1/2 cup of barbecue sauce
- 2 tablespoons of red onion finely chopped
- 20 frozen large-sized raw shrimp, peeled & deveined 26 to 30 per pound
- 1 tablespoon of fresh cilantro chopped
- 2 teaspoons of lime juice
- 2 teaspoons of freshly grated ginger
- 1 tablespoon of finely chopped & seeded jalapeño
- 1/2 cup of brown rice uncooked
- 1 cup of chopped fresh mango
- 1 medium mango

Instructions:

Follow the instructions below to make BBQ shrimps with tropical rice. Thaw shrimp as directed on the box.

1. Prepare brown rice as directed on the package, eliminating salt; set aside.
2. In the meantime, thread the shrimp onto Four metal skewers, allowing 1/8-inch between each shrimp. Combine the barbecue sauce & ginger in a small-sized mixing dish. Grill shrimp for 6 to 7 minutes on an oiled rack of an uncovered grill directly on medium heat, rotating once and coating with sauce mixture constantly.

3. In a large-sized mixing bowl, combine the mango, onion, jalapeno, cilantro, and lime juice. Serve immediately on serving plates. Serve the shrimp over the rice.

Salmon with Cranberry Chutney Glazed

Cooking time: 10 minutes

Preparation time: 10 minutes

Servings: 4

Per serving: Calories 229, Total fat 9g, Protein 28g, Carbs 7g

Ingredients:

- 1/2 teaspoon of ground cinnamon
- 1/4 cup of cranberry chutney
- 1/2 teaspoon of salt optional
- 4 salmon fillets skinless around 5 to 6 ounces each
- 1 tablespoon of white wine vinegar
- 1/4 teaspoon of ground red pepper

Instructions:

Follow the instructions below to make salmon with cranberry chutney glazed.

1. Preheat the broiler or have the grill ready for indirect grilling. In a small-sized cup, combine cinnamon, salt, and ground red pepper; sprinkle over fish. In a small-sized bowl, combine the chutney & vinegar; brush a tiny quantity equally across each salmon fillet.
2. Broil around 5 to 6 inches from the heat source or grill 4 to 6 minutes on medium-hot coals on a covered grill till salmon is opaque in the middle.

Prawn and Avocado Cocktails

Cooking time: 0 minutes

Preparation time: 10 minutes

Servings: 4

Per serving: Calories 302, Total fat 28g, Protein 3g, Carbs 13g

Ingredients:

For the dressing:

- 1 orange juice
- 4 tablespoons of olive oil

For the salad:

- 1 finely chopped avocado
- 2 finely sliced spring onions
- 1 finely chopped fennel bulb
- Salt & pepper to taste
- 2 large finely chopped tomatoes
- 200 g of cooked prawns

Instructions:

Follow the instructions below to make prawn and avocado cocktails.

1. To make the dressing: combine the olive oil & orange juice in a bowl and set aside.
2. For the salad: In a large-sized mixing bowl, combine the chopped fennel, prawns, tomatoes, avocado, and spring onions.
3. Before serving, distribute the salad among Four Martini glasses & drizzle with the dressing.

Peppery Flavor COD with Mixed Veggies

Cooking time: 20 minutes

Preparation time: 10 minutes

Servings: 4

Per serving: Calories 606, Total fat 14g, Protein 78g, Carbs 12g

Ingredients:

- 8 x 200 g of cod fillets
- 500 g of asparagus
- Salt & freshly ground pepper to taste
- 100 g of sun-dried tomatoes
- 3 tablespoons of olive oil

Instructions:

Follow the instructions below to make peppery flavor COD with mixed veggies. At 400°F, preheat the oven.

1. Set aside the asparagus after steaming it for 3 minutes.
2. Season the cod fillets on both sides with salt and set them on a baking tray. Bake for around 15 minutes after drizzling with olive oil.
3. On a bed of mixed salad & sun-dried tomatoes, arrange the cod fillets with asparagus. Serve the fish immediately after seasoning it with freshly ground pepper.

Grilled Basil Flavor Shrimps

Cooking time: 10 minutes

Preparation time: 15 minutes

Servings: 4

Per serving: Calories 180, Total fat 8g, Protein 24g, Carbs 3g

Ingredients:
- 1 ounce of minced fresh basil approximately 1 cup
- 1/2 large lemon juice
- A pinch of black pepper
- 1 tablespoon of olive oil
- Cooking spray
- 1 1/2 tablespoons of reduced-calorie melted margarine
- 1 clove of minced garlic
- 1 tablespoon of coarse-grain prepared mustard
- 1 pound of medium-sized fresh shrimp, peeled & deveined

Instructions:

Follow the instructions below to make grilled basil flavor shrimps.

1. Whisk together margarine, olive oil, lemon juice, garlic, mustard, basil, and pepper in a small- sized bowl; transfer to a large zip-top bag. Toss in the shrimp & gently toss to coat. Refrigerate for 1 hour to marinate. Heat the grill to medium-high. Remove the shrimp from the marinade & skewer them. Spray the grill grate with nonstick cooking spray. Place the skewers on the grill on medium-high flame and drizzle with any leftover marinade. Cook for around 2 to 3 minutes, then flip the shrimp and cook for another 2–3 minutes, or until pink and opaque. Chilled or reheated leftovers are both acceptable options.

Tasty Salmon with Basil Sauce

Cooking time: 15 minutes

Preparation time: 10 minutes

Servings: 4

Per serving: Calories 274, Total fat 21g, Protein 19g, Carbs 4g

Ingredients:

- 200 g of fresh basil
- Salt & ground black pepper to taste
- 4 salmon steaks approx. 200 g each
- 2 lemons juice
- 5 tablespoons of olive oil

Instructions:

Follow the instructions below to make tasty salmon with basil sauce.

1. Pull the basil leaves out of their stalks & pulse them in a food processor until smooth.
2. Add the lemon juice as well as a pinch of salt and black pepper to taste. Slowly drizzle in the olive oil & set aside.
3. Brush the steaks with olive oil and cook for 10 minutes on a barbecue or grill. Enjoy with the basil sauce on the side.

Tamarind Flavor Prawns

Cooking time: 20 minutes

Preparation time: 10 minutes

Servings: 4

Per serving: Calories 611, Total fat 16g, Protein 32g, Carbs 86g

Ingredients:

- 2 tablespoons of agave nectar
- 500 g of shelled prawns
- 200 ml of water
- 800 g of cooked soba noodles
- 30 g of tamarind paste available in all good supermarkets
- 2 finely sliced shallots
- 5 tablespoons of vegetable oil
- 3 chopped spring onions
- 1finely chopped small onion
- 4 finely chopped garlic cloves

Instructions:

Follow the instructions below to make tamarind flavor prawns.

1. Bring a large saucepan of water to a boil, then put the soba noodles and cook in the simmering water for 5 minutes.
2. Fill a pan halfway with water & bring it to a boil.
3. Pour the boiling water over the tamarind paste in a bowl.
4. Make sure there are also no lumps in the tamarind sauce by completely mixing it. Set aside for 30 minutes.
5. In a wok over high heat, heat the oil & add the onion. Cook the onion until it turns golden brown, about 3 minutes.
6. Combine the agave nectar, water, and tamarind paste. Put this mixture to a boil after thoroughly mixing it.
7. Stir in the shallots, garlic, & prawns for around 3 minutes.

8. Place the prawns on a bed of soba noodles with spring onions on top!

Tasty COD with Sautéed Kale

Cooking time: 25 minutes

Preparation time: 5 minutes

Servings: 4

Per serving: Calories 380, Total fat 1g, Protein 33g, Carbs 19g

Ingredients:

For the fish:

- 2 teaspoons of chopped thyme leaves
- 4 x 170 g of cod fillets
- 1/2 chopped red bell pepper
- 1 tablespoon of fresh lemon juice
- 400 g of finely chopped tinned tomatoes
- 1 teaspoon of lemon zest
- Himalayan sea salt & black pepper, to taste

For the kale:

- 1tablespoon of red wine vinegar
- 450 g of kale, tough stems & ribs removed & cut into 1-inch strips
- Dash of sea salt
- 2 tablespoons of olive oil

Instructions:

Follow the instructions below to make tasty COD with sautéed kale.

1. At 400°F, preheat the oven.
2. Coconut oil should be lightly sprayed or coated on a 13x9" 33x23cm oven tray.
3. Mix the tomatoes, peppers, salt, lemon zest, thyme, and pepper in a saucepan. Cook for 5 minutes or until soft.

4. Season the fish with a touch of salt and black pepper and place it in the prepared baking dish. Bake for around 10 minutes in a preheated oven.
5. One tablespoon of lemon juice should be drizzled on top.
6. To make the kale: 1/2 a saucepan of water is brought to a boil, then the kale is added. Bring the kale to a boil for about 10 minutes.
7. Remove the kale from flame and set it aside to drain. Heat a bit of oil to a medium-high temperature.
8. Cook for around 1 minute, or until the garlic softens.
9. 1Reduce flame to a low setting and stir in the kale. Simmer, occasionally stirring, until the contents of the pan are thoroughly warmed.
10. 1Remove the pan from the flame and add the vinegar & salt.
11. Serve the fish with the veggie mixture on the side, on a bed of kale.

Easy and Quick Salmon & Tomato Twangs

Cooking time: 15 minutes

Preparation time: 5 minutes

Servings: 4

Per serving: Calories 393, Total fat 24g, Protein 46g, Carbs 1g

Ingredients:

- 1 teaspoon of finely chopped parsley
- 2 tablespoons of lemon juice
- 4 fresh salmon fillets
- 1 teaspoon of finely chopped basil
- 6 finely chopped medium-sized tomatoes
- Salt and black pepper to taste
- 1 teaspoon of finely chopped coriander

Instructions:

Follow the instructions below to make easy and quick salmon and tomato twangs.

1. In a bowl, combine the herbs, tomatoes, and lemon juice.
2. Make a thorough mix.
3. Place the salmon fillets on a prepared baking pan, skin side up, at 360°F in a preheated oven. Season the tomato mixture and place on top of the salmon before baking for 15 minutes.

Prawn Salad with Asparagus

Cooking time: 5 minutes

Preparation time: 10 minutes

Servings: 4

Per serving: Calories 219, Total fat 16g, Protein 3g, Carbs 1g

Ingredients:

- 80 ml of extra-virgin olive oil
- 1 lemon juice
- 400 g of woody stems removed asparagus
- 1 tablespoon of finely chopped fresh parsley
- Salt & black pepper to taste
- 220 g of cooked king prawns
- 1 finely chopped garlic clove

Instructions:

Follow the instructions below to make a prawn salad with asparagus.

1. In a medium-sized saucepan, bring some water to a boil.
2. Add asparagus and boil; after 3 minutes of boiling, asparagus Drain the asparagus and set it aside.
3. Cook the prawns for 30 seconds in boiling water. In a large-sized mixing dish, place the prawns.
4. Place the asparagus spears in the bowl with prawns after slicing them. Mix in the remaining ingredients in a mixing bowl.

Flavorsome Zingy Whole Mackerel

Cooking time: 10 minutes

Preparation time: 10 minutes

Servings: 4

Per serving: Calories 256, Total fat 18g, Protein 20.5g, Carbs 5g

Ingredients:

- 4 teaspoons of finely chopped garlic
- Juice and zest of 2 limes
- 4 whole mackerel, gutted & cleaned
- 1 teaspoon of Thai fish sauce
- 4 teaspoons of finely chopped ginger
- 2 tablespoons of sesame oil
- 1 large-sized red chili, deseeded & chopped

Instructions:

Follow the instructions below to make flavorsome zingy whole mackerel.

1. Wash the mackerel, score both sides 5 or 6 times, and be careful not to strike the bone. Stir the sesame oil, lime zest and juice, garlic, ginger, chili, and Thai fish sauce in a mixing dish.
2. Apply the marinade to each mackerel.
3. Grill the mackerel for about 5 minutes on each side, or until it is browned and the eyes are white.
4. Place the fish in a large dish with any remaining marinade and season to taste, then set aside for 3 minutes before serving with a side salad.

Crab, Artichoke and Spinach Dip

Cooking time: 30 minutes

Preparation time: 0 minutes

Servings: 10

Per serving: Calories 99, Total fat 7g, Protein 6g, Carbs 3g

Ingredients:

- 1/4 teaspoon of hot pepper sauce
- 1 can of 6 1/2 ounces crabmeat, drained & shredded
- 1 package 8 ounces of low-fat cream cheese
- Melba toast or whole-grain crackers optional
- 1 package 10 ounces of frozen and chopped spinach, thawed and squeezed nearly dry
- 1 jar about 6 ounces of marinated artichoke hearts, drained & finely chopped

Instructions:

Follow the instructions below to make crab, artichoke and spinach dip.

1. Remove any shell and cartilage from the crabmeat and discard. In a 1 1/2-quart slow cooker, add crabmeat, artichokes, spinach, cream cheese, and hot pepper sauce.
2. Cook, covered, on high for 30 minutes or until thoroughly cooked. If desired, serve with melba toast.

Southern-Style Crab Cakes with Dipping Sauce

Cooking time: 15 minutes

Preparation time: 10 minutes

Servings: 8

Per serving: Calories 81, Total fat 2g, Protein 7g, Carbs 8g

Ingredients:

- 1/4 cup of green onions chopped
- 2 teaspoons of olive oil, divided
- 10 ounces of fresh lump crabmeat
- 1 lightly beaten egg white
- 3/4 teaspoon of hot pepper sauce, divided
- 1 1/2 cups of fresh white or sourdough bread crumbs, divided
- 1/2 cup of fat-free or low-fat mayonnaise, divided
- Lemon wedges optional
- 2 tablespoons of coarse-grained or spicy brown mustard, divided

Instructions:

Follow the instructions below to make Southern-style crab cakes with dipping sauce.

1. At 200°F, preheat the oven. Remove any shell from the crabmeat and discard. In a medium- sized mixing bowl, combine 3/4 cup bread crumbs, crabmeat, and green onions. Mix together 1/4 cup mayonnaise, 1 tablespoon of mustard, & 1/2 teaspoon of hot pepper sauce. Form 8 1/2-inch- thick cakes with 1/4 cup of the mixture each cake. Roll the crab cakes in the leftover 3/4 cup of bread crumbs lightly.
2. Put 1 teaspoon of oil, heat in a large-sized nonstick skillet on medium flame. Cook the cakes for around 4 to 5 minutes per side or till golden brown, adding 4 crab cakes at a time. Place

on a serving plate and keep warm in the oven. Repeat with the crab cakes and the remaining 1 teaspoon oil.

3. In a separate dish, whisk together the remaining 1/4 cup of mayonnaise, 1 tablespoon of mustard, & 1/4 teaspoon of hot pepper sauce for the dipping sauce.

4. If desired, serve warm crab cakes with dipping sauce & lemon wedges.

Tasty Thai-Style Fennel Tuna

Cooking time: 15 minutes

Preparation time: 10 minutes

Servings: 4

Per serving: Calories 330, Total fat 4g, Protein 39g, Carbs 19g

Ingredients:

- 2 tablespoons of olive oil
- 4 tuna steaks, around 140g of each
- Salt & pepper to taste
- 2 thickly sliced lengthways fennel bulbs
- For the marinade:
- 2 lemon juice and zest
- 125 ml of extra virgin olive oil
- 4 fresh red chilies, deseeded & finely chopped
- 4 tablespoons of finely chopped fresh parsley
- 4 garlic cloves finely chopped

Instructions:

Follow the instructions below to make tasty Thai-style fennel tuna.

1. In a small-sized mixing dish, combine all of the marinade ingredients.
2. Place the tuna steaks in a large and shallow dish & pour 4 tablespoons of marinade over them, turning to coat well.
3. Cover and marinate for approximately 30 minutes in the refrigerator. Save the rest of the marinade for another time.
4. On high flame, heat a ridged griddle pan.
5. Place the fennel into the pan and pour the oil over it. Cook for 5 minutes on each side, or until color appears. Then divide over four hot serving dishes.
6. Cook the tuna steaks in the griddle pan for 4 to 5 minutes on each side, or until firm to the touch but still wet inside.

7. On each serving plate, arrange the tuna on top of the fennel & sprinkle with the leftover marinade.

Classic Fish Pie

Cooking time: 25 minutes

Preparation time: 5 minutes

Servings: 2

Per serving: Calories 409, Total fat 20.3g, Protein 19g, Carbs 20.5g

Ingredients:
- 2 garlic cloves
- 1/2 teaspoon of ground ginger
- 120 g of salmon
- 2 tablespoons of olive oil
- 1/2 teaspoon of cinnamon
- 140 g of smoked haddock
- 1 finely chopped onion
- 1x 400 g tin of chopped tomatoes
- Salt & pepper
- For the mash:
- 300 g of carrots
- 25 g of butter
- Salt & pepper
- 300 g of celeriac

Instructions:

Follow the instructions below to make classic fish pie. At 350°F, preheat the oven.

1. Boil the celeriac & carrots for 8 to 10 minutes in salted water. Using a strainer, mash and stir in the butter. To taste, season with salt & pepper.
2. Place the fish in a pot with just enough water to cover it and bring to a boil and cook for around 5 minutes.
3. The fish should flake easily and become opaque. Place the fish in a bowl after draining it.

4. In a medium-sized saucepan, heat the oil and sauté the garlic and onions for 5 minutes. Combine the cooked fish, ginger, chopped tomatoes, cinnamon, and salt and black pepper. Allow the flavor to penetrate by simmering on a medium flame.
5. Fill a small roasting tin halfway with the mixture and top with the mash. Cook for around 15 minutes in the oven or until the mash becomes crunchy. 1Serve with a vegetable side dish, a green salad, or by itself.

Delicious COD Parsley Parcels

Cooking time: 25 minutes

Preparation time: 5 minutes

Servings: 4

Per serving: Calories 230, Total fat 6g, Protein 32g, Carbs 1g

Ingredients:

- 3 tablespoons of finely chopped fresh parsley
- 4 cod fillets, approx. 170g of each, skinned
- 1 tablespoon of plain flour
- Salt & pepper to taste
- 2 teaspoons of butter
- 500 ml of semi-skimmed milk
- 2 tablespoons of lemon juice

Instructions:

Follow the instructions below to make delicious COD parsley parcels.

1. Bring the milk to a boil with the lemon juice, salt, and black pepper. Allow 30 minutes to cool after boiling.
2. Melt the butter in a small-sized saucepan on low flame, then stir in the flour until smooth. Cook for around a minute after stirring.
3. Slowly drizzle in the milk, whisking continually.
4. Return to the flame and bring to a boil, stirring constantly.
5. Boil for around 10 minutes, then season to taste with salt and black pepper.
6. Put the cod fillets inside the pan & poach for 4–6 minutes on low flame, without allowing the sauce to boil, until the fish is done.
7. After 2 minutes, flip each piece of fish.

8. Put the fish fillets on a serving platter & pour the parsley sauce over them.

Chicken And Poultry Recipes

Grilled Chicken with Black Beans and Corn Salsa

Cooking time: 15 minutes

Preparation time: 10 minutes

Servings: 4

Per serving: Calories 230, Total fat 7g, Protein 30g, Carbs 16g

Ingredients:

- 1/2 cup of red bell pepper finely chopped
- 2 tablespoons of fresh lime juice
- 1/2 ripe medium diced avocado
- 1/2 teaspoon of salt, divided
- 4 boneless and skinless chicken breasts about 4 ounces each, pounded into 1/2-inch thickness
- 1/2 cup of corn
- 1/4 cup of fresh cilantro chopped
- Nonstick cooking spray
- 1/2 15-ounces can of black beans, rinsed & drained
- 1 teaspoon of black pepper
- 1 tablespoon of chopped, sliced and pickled jalapeño pepper
- 1/2 teaspoon of chili powder

Instructions:

Follow the instructions below to make grilled chicken with black beans and corn salsa.

1. In a medium-sized mixing bowl, combine corn, bell pepper, beans, jalapeno, avocado, cilantro, lime juice, & 1/4 teaspoon of salt. Set them aside.
2. In a small dish, combine the black pepper, remaining 1/4 of teaspoon salt, & chili powder; sprinkle over chicken.
3. Spray the grill pan with nonstick cooking spray. Cook chicken for 4 minutes per side on a medium-high flame, or till no longer pink in the middle.

4. Serve chicken with half of the salsa on top; keep the leftover salsa refrigerated for another time.

Tasty Grilled South of the Border Chicken

Cooking time: 20 minutes

Preparation time: 5 minutes

Servings: 4

Per serving: Calories 201, Total fat 7g, Protein 26g, Carbs 5g

Ingredients:

- 2 teaspoons of lemon juice
- 4 small skinless and boneless chicken breasts
- 1/2 cup of low-fat sour cream
- 1 packet of taco seasoning search for reduced-sodium taco seasoning.

Instructions:

Follow the instructions below to make tasty grilled south of the border chicken.

1. With a wire whisk, combine lemon juice, sour cream, and taco seasoning in a medium- sized bowl.
2. Clean the chicken breasts by rinsing them and patting them dry. Coat chicken breasts equally in sour cream mixture.
3. Grill the breasts for 10 minutes per side or till cooked through. Serve the food. If you don't have access to a grill, you may cook the chicken breasts in a skillet sprayed with nonstick cooking spray on medium to medium-low flame on the stovetop.

Simple and Quick Lemon Chicken

Cooking time: 25 minutes

Preparation time: 5 minutes

Servings: 4

Per serving: Calories 195, Total fat 7g, Protein 30g, Carbs 3g

Ingredients:
- 1 tablespoon of olive oil
- Nonstick cooking spray
- 1/2 teaspoon white pepper
- 1 pound of boneless and skinless chicken breast 4 pieces
- 1/2 teaspoon of onion powder
- 1 1/2 teaspoons of oregano
- 1 large-sized lemon

Instructions:

Follow the instructions below to make simple and quick lemon chicken.

1. At 375°F, preheat the oven. Tear out a large enough sheet of aluminum foil to wrap all 4 pieces of chicken with. Spray the aluminum foil on one side only using nonstick cooking spray and place the chicken breasts on it. Drizzle with extra virgin olive oil. Grate one tablespoon of lemon zest, grated, keep it aside. Remove the seeds from the lemon before juicing it. Coat chicken with lemon zest, white pepper, onion powder, and oregano after pouring lemon juice over it. To construct a sealed packet, fold the aluminum foil all over the chicken & roll the edges together. In a jelly roll pan or a large, shallow casserole dish, place the packet. Bake 25 minutes in the oven. Remove the chicken from the oven & carefully open the foil with tongs to transfer it to a serving platter.

Crispy Chicken Nuggets with BBQ Dipping Sauce

Cooking time: 15 minutes

Preparation time: 10 minutes

Servings: 8

Per serving: Calories 167, Total fat 4g, Protein 14g, Carbs 16g

Ingredients:
- 1/4 cup of almond flour
- 1 teaspoon of dried oregano
- 1 pound of boneless and skinless chicken breasts
- Dash of black pepper
- 3 tablespoons of barbecue sauce
- 1/4 teaspoon of salt
- 2 tablespoons of peach or apricot fruit spread no-sugar-added
- 1 egg white
- 2 cups of crushed reduced-fat baked cheese crackers
- 1 tablespoon of water

Instructions:

Follow the instructions below to make crispy chicken nuggets with BBQ dipping sauce.

2. At 400°F, preheat the oven. Chicken should be cut into Forty 1-inch pieces.
3. In a large-sized resealable food storage bag, combine flour, salt, & pepper. In a small- sized bowl, combine cracker crumbs & oregano. In another small-sized bowl, whisk together the egg white & water.
4. Add chicken pieces in a bag with the flour mixture and seal. Shake until all of the chicken is evenly coated. Take the chicken out of the bag and shake off any excess flour. Coat the chicken pieces on all sides with the egg white mixture. Roll the dough in the crumb mixture. Place in a baking pan with a shallow bottom. Rep with the rest of the chicken

pieces. Bake for around 10 to 13 minutes, or till golden brown.

5. Meanwhile, in a small-sized saucepan, combine the barbecue sauce & jam; continue cooking on low heat until thoroughly cooked. Serve the chicken nuggets with a dipping sauce on the side.

Roasted Chopped Chicken Salad

Cooking time: 20 minutes

Preparation time: 10 minutes

Servings: 4

Per serving: Calories 253, Total fat 9g, Protein 29g, Carbs 15g

Ingredients:

- 1 teaspoon of balsamic vinegar
- 6 cups of romaine lettuce chopped
- 1/2 cup of chopped and drained artichoke hearts
- 2 cloves of minced garlic
- 1/2 cup of canned cannellini beans, rinsed & drained
- 1 teaspoon of dried basil
- 1/4 teaspoon of red pepper flakes
- 1/2 cup of quartered red or yellow grape tomatoes
- 1/2 cup of balsamic vinaigrette dressing low-fat
- 2 bone-in and skin-on chicken breasts
- 1/2 cup of chopped and roasted red peppers
- 2 cups of chopped baby arugula

Instructions:

Follow the instructions below to make roasted chopped chicken salad.

1. At 400°F, preheat the oven. On a rimmed baking sheet, place a wire rack.
2. In a large-sized serving bowl, combine lettuce, arugula, beans, tomatoes, artichoke hearts, roasted peppers, as well as the remaining chicken. Serve with a side of dressing.
3. In a small-sized bowl, combine the vinegar, garlic, basil, and red pepper flakes. Spread half of the garlic mixture under the skin of each chicken breast with care. Place the chicken on a wire rack to cool. Roast for 20 minutes, or until the center is

no longer pink. Remove the skin and set it aside until it is safe to handle. Chop the chicken and set aside 1/2 cup for another recipe.

Chicken with Artichokes and Spinach

Cooking time: 25 minutes

Preparation time: 5 minutes

Servings: 2

Per serving: Calories 328, Total fat 11g, Protein 37g, Carbs 19g

Ingredients:

- 4 canned artichoke hearts, drained & chopped
- 1 cup of frozen chopped spinach, thawed & well-drained
- 1/4 cup of frozen chopped onions, thawed & well-drained
- 1 cup of chopped and cooked chicken pieces
- 1/4 cup + 2 tablespoons of grated Parmesan cheese, divided
- 1/8 teaspoon of black pepper
- 1/2 teaspoon of minced garlic
- 1/4 cup of fat-free mayonnaise

Instructions:

Follow the instructions below to make chicken with artichokes and spinach.

1. At 375°F, preheat the oven. Using nonstick cooking spray, coat a 1-quart casserole.
2. In a medium-sized mixing bowl, combine spinach, artichoke hearts, 2 tablespoons of cheese, garlic, onions, mayonnaise, and pepper. Place the chicken in the prepared casserole & equally distribute the spinach mixture on top. Add the remaining 1/4 cup of cheese on top.
3. Bake for around 25 minutes or until the cheese is golden brown.

Chicken Salad with Spinach

Cooking time: 5 minutes

Preparation time: 15 minutes

Servings: 4

Per serving: Calories 218, Total fat 4g, Protein 23g, Carbs 4g

Ingredients:

- 2 cups of washed & torn romaine lettuce
- 3/4 pound of chicken tenders
- 1/4 cup of fat-free Italian salad dressing prepared
- Nonstick cooking spray
- 8 thin slices of red onion, separated into rings
- 4 cups of shredded stemmed spinach
- Assorted fresh greens optional
- 1 large-sized grapefruit, peeled & sectioned
- 2 tablespoons of crumbled blue cheese

Instructions:

Follow the instructions below to make chicken salad with spinach.

1. Chicken should be cut into 2 1/2-inch strips. Cook on medium flame in a large-sized nonstick skillet sprayed with cooking spray. Cook & stir for 5 minutes, or until the chicken is no longer pink in the middle. Remove the pan from the flame. Distribute spinach, cheese, lettuce, grapefruit, onion, & chicken between 4 salad plates, combine the citrus blend concentrate & the Italian dressing, sprinkle over salads.

Pepper-Lemon Chicken Wings

Cooking time: 25 minutes

Preparation time: 5 minutes

Servings: 4

Per serving: Calories 291, Total fat 20g, Protein 27g, Carbs 2g

Ingredients:

- 2 pounds of free-range chicken wings
- 1 tablespoon of freshly ground black pepper
- Large-sized baking sheet, lined with foil, with the wire rack set on top
- 2 tablespoons of freshly squeezed lemon juice
- 1 teaspoon of sea salt
- 2 tablespoons of grated lemon zest

Instructions:

Follow the instructions below to make pepper-lemon chicken wings.

1. Remove as much moisture as possible from the chicken by patting it dry with paper towels. Place on the wire rack over the baking sheet that has been prepared, leaving space between them if feasible.
2. Roast for around 25 minutes in a preheated oven, rotating halfway through, till juices run clear whenever pierced.
3. Meanwhile, add lemon zest, pepper, lemon juice, & salt in a large-sized mixing dish. Toss the wings in the lemon sauce until they are uniformly coated. Serve immediately.

Fajita Flavor Grilled Chicken

Cooking time: 10 minutes

Preparation time: 5 minutes

Servings: 2

Per serving: Calories 176, Total fat 8g, Protein 19g, Carbs 8g

Ingredients:
- 1 bunch of green onions, ends trimmed
- 2 teaspoons of fajita seasoning mix
- 2 boneless and skinless chicken breasts around 4 ounces each
- 1 tablespoon of olive oil

Instructions:

Follow the instructions below to make fajita flavor grilled chicken. Get your grill ready for direct cooking.

1. Drizzle oil over the chicken & green onions. Season chicken breasts on both sides with a spice mix. Cook 6 to 8 minutes on the grill, or till chicken is no pinker in the center.
2. Toss the chicken with the onions and serve.

Dinner Chicken Salad with a Green Onion Dressing

Cooking time: 25 minutes

Preparation time: 5 minutes

Servings: 4

Per serving: Calories 255, Total fat 15g, Protein 18g, Carbs 12g

Ingredients:
- 1 large sliced thinly cucumber about 8 inches
- 4 cooked chicken breasts 3 ounces each, boneless and skinless
- 1 teaspoon of Worcestershire sauce
- 1/4 teaspoon of black pepper
- 4 cups of iceberg lettuce, washed & torn into bite-size pieces
- 2 packets of Splenda
- 4 small-sized tomatoes around 3 1/2 inches in diameter
- 1/4 cup of extra-virgin olive oil
- 2 dashes of salt
- 1 cup of grated carrot
- 1 teaspoon of dry mustard
- 1/4 cup of fresh cilantro leaves optional
- 4 ounces of green onions
- 1/3 cup of red wine vinegar
- 2 tablespoons of water

Instructions:

Follow the instructions below to make dinner chicken salad with a green onion dressing.

1. Set aside the chicken, which has been cut into bite-size cubes. On each of the four salad plates, put 1 cup of torn iceberg lettuce. Each tomato should be quartered and placed around each plate. On each dish, evenly distribute cucumber slices between tomato slices. Grated carrots around 1/4 cup each plate and chicken are served on top.

2. Trim the green onions' roots & 2 inches from the tops. Combine all of the dressing ingredients in a food processor or blender and pulse until well combined. Around 1/4 cup dressing should be poured over each salad. If desired, garnish with cilantro.

Chicken Kiev's Stuffed with Feta and Spinach

Cooking time: 20 minutes

Preparation time: 10 minutes

Servings: 2

Per serving: Calories 772, Total fat 41g, Protein 60g, Carbs 7g

Ingredients:

- 200 g of fresh spinach Rocket & watercress
- 2 teaspoons of red wine vinegar for salad dressing
- 4 chicken breasts boneless, around 600g
- 2 tablespoons of pine nuts
- Sea salt & freshly ground black pepper, to taste
- 8 slices of Parma ham
- 120 g of crumbled feta cheese
- 2 tablespoons of olive oil

Instructions:

Follow the instructions below to make chicken Kiev's stuffed with feta and spinach.

1. At 380°F, preheat the oven.
2. In a saucepan on medium flame, toast the pine nuts for around 3 to 4 minutes, then set aside.
3. Put the spinach in a skillet & simmer for 2 to 3 minutes, frequently stirring, until it wilts. Remove the pan from the flame & set it aside to cool for a few minutes. Drain the spinach & press out as much liquid as possible with your hands or in a colander.
4. Coarsely chop the spinach with a big knife & transfer it to a small-sized bowl. Stir in the feta & pine nuts until everything is well combined. Season with salt & freshly ground black pepper.

5. Each chicken breast should have a little pocket cut into it. Fill each pocket with the spinach mixture. To enclose the filling, wrap two slices of Parma ham around each one.
6. Put the chicken on a baking pan and bake for around 20 minutes in a preheated oven.
7. In a small bowl/cup, combine the olive oil & red wine vinegar and pour over the rocket & watercress.
8. Serve 2 Kiev's with the dressed rocket & watercress salad on a dinner platter.

Tempting Sticky Chicken

Cooking time: 25 minutes

Preparation time: 5 minutes

Servings: 4

Per serving: Calories 385, Total fat 18g, Protein 44g, Carbs 9g

Ingredients:

- 6 chicken thighs
- 6 chicken drumsticks
- For the marinade:
- 2 tablespoons of agave nectar
- 1 tablespoon of finely chopped ginger
- 1 finely chopped green chili
- 3 tablespoons of light soy sauce
- Juice of 1 lemon
- 3 teaspoons of ground allspice
- 6 finely chopped garlic cloves

Instructions:

Follow the instructions below to make tempting sticky chicken.

1. In a large-sized mixing bowl, combine the soy sauce, agave nectar, allspice, lemon juice, garlic, ginger, & chili.
2. Slit the chicken & pour the marinade inside. Refrigerate the chicken overnight, covered in cling film.
3. At 450°F, preheat the oven.
4. After that put the chicken in a roasting pan. Pour the remaining marinade over the chicken and bake it in the oven for about 20 minutes.
5. When the chicken is sticky and golden, it's done. Serve with homemade coleslaw to round up the meal.

Chicken Mushroom and Cashew Nut Risotto

Cooking time: 25 minutes

Preparation time: 5 minutes

Servings: 4

Per serving: Calories 494, Total fat 26g, Protein 26g, Carbs 49g

Ingredients:

- 25 g of pine nuts
- 4l of hot vegetable stock
- 2 tablespoons of olive oil
- Salt & freshly ground pepper to taste
- 200 g of risotto rice
- 250 g of cooked chicken
- 30 g of butter
- 100 g of large mushrooms
- 2 spring onions
- 30 g of cashew nuts

Instructions:

Follow the instructions below to make chicken mushroom and cashew nut risotto.

1. In a large-sized saucepan on medium flame, combine the olive oil & butter.
2. After the butter has melted, add the spring garlic and spring onions and sauté for another 2 minutes. Finally, add the rice & toss it around to evenly coat everything.
3. Cook the rice for around 10 minutes after adding half of the stock.
4. Cook for yet another 10 minutes, frequently stirring, until the rice is soft and creamy, adding the rest of the stock, mushrooms, and cashew nuts.
5. Take the pan off the flame and add the chicken & pine nuts.

6. Salt & freshly ground pepper the risotto generously. Put it on a plate and savor it!

Thai-Style Chicken Satay

Cooking time: 15 minutes

Preparation time: 10 minutes

Servings: 4

Per serving: Calories 478, Total fat 23g, Protein 59g, Carbs 5g

Ingredients:

- 1 small finely chopped white onion
- 50 g of raw peanuts, shelled & skinned
- 2 finely chopped garlic cloves
- 4 tablespoons of crunchy peanut butter
- 5 tablespoons of vegetable oil
- 600 g of chicken breast, slice into 1/2 inch by 2-inch pieces
- 1 tablespoon of soy sauce
- 2 teaspoons of finely chopped ginger
- 2 tablespoons of chili sauce

Instructions:

Follow the instructions below to make Thai-style chicken satay.

1. Cut the peanuts into little pieces with a diameter of around 12 centimeters. In a wok, heat 1/2 tablespoon of the vegetable oil.
2. Stir fry the peanuts for about a minute till golden brown in the heated oil. Drain on kitchen paper after removing with a slotted spoon.
3. In the same pan, heat the remaining oil and add the onion, ginger, & garlic once it's hot. Stir- fry for 2 minutes using this combination.
4. Add chicken and stir fry for about 3 minutes, or until the chicken pieces are crisp and brown on all sides.
5. Using bamboo skewers, thread the chicken.

6. Serve as a dipping sauce by combining the crunchy peanut butter, chill sauce, & soy sauce.

Tasty Chicken with Asparagus

Cooking time: 15 minutes

Preparation time: 10 minutes

Servings: 4

Per serving: Calories 299, Total fat 5g, Protein 31g, Carbs 9g

Ingredients:

- 4 small onions, peeled & chopped into 1-inch pieces
- 1 teaspoon of chili-garlic sauce
- 500 g of fresh asparagus, hard ends trimmed, chopped into 1-inch pieces
- 1 tablespoon of toasted sesame oil
- 450 g of skinless chicken breast fillets, diced
- 1 tablespoon of ginger, peeled & finely chopped
- 2 tablespoons of vegetable oil
- 1 tablespoon of oyster sauce

Instructions:

Follow the instructions below to make tasty chicken with asparagus.

1. In a medium-sized pan, heat the vegetable oil.
2. Add the chicken pieces in the hot oil & cook, stirring regularly, for about 7 minutes, or until white on all sides.
3. In a wok on a high flame, heat the sesame oil.
4. Cook for an additional minute with the asparagus before adding the prepared chicken.
5. Finally, add the ginger, onions, oyster sauce, & chili-garlic sauce, and cook for 3 minutes before serving.

Thai-Style Green Chicken Curry

Cooking time: 25 minutes

Preparation time: 5 minutes

Servings: 2

Per serving: Calories 409, Total fat 20.3g, Protein 19g, Carbs 20.5g

Ingredients:

- 4 finely chopped spring onions
- 2 chicken breasts
- 1 tablespoon of coconut oil
- 1/2 teaspoon of coriander seeds
- 2 finely chopped garlic cloves
- 5 cm piece of finely grated fresh ginger
- 2 teaspoons of fish sauce
- 100 g of bean sprouts
- 400 ml of coconut milk
- 1 sliced medium white onion
- 5 g of Thai green curry paste
- Chopped fresh coriander
- 1 stick of finely chopped lemongrass
- 1 lemon juice and zest
- 1 green chili deseeded & sliced
- 1/2 teaspoon of cumin seeds

Instructions:

Follow the instructions below to make Thai-style green chicken curry.

1. Chicken breasts should be cut into small pieces.
2. In a nonstick wok, heat the coconut oil on low to medium flame.

3. Cook for 4 to 5 minutes with the chicken, onions, ginger, garlic, lemongrass, and chili. In a pestle and mortar, grind the coriander & cumin seeds.
4. To infuse the chicken, put these into the wok.
5. Combine the Thai green curry paste, fish sauce, coconut milk, lime juice and zest, and 1/2 of the fresh coriander.
6. Simmer the mixture for 15 minutes on medium flame.
7. Finally, put the bean sprouts & the remaining coriander, and cook for another five minutes on high heat.
8. Serve right away with a squeeze of lime juice on top to taste.

Simple Fried Chicken

Cooking time: 25 minutes

Preparation time: 5 minutes

Servings: 6

Per serving: Calories 282, Total fat 21g, Protein 15g, Carbs 2g

Ingredients:

- 120 g of ground almonds
- 1/2 teaspoon of dried parsley
- 1/2 teaspoon of dried sage
- Salt & pepper to taste
- 6 skin-on chicken drumsticks
- 1/4 teaspoon of Chinese five-spice
- 1 teaspoon of paprika
- 1/2 teaspoon of ginger powder
- 2 tablespoons of olive oil
- 1/4 teaspoon of chili powder
- 1/2 teaspoon of mustard powder
- 1/2 teaspoon of dried basil

Instructions:

Follow the instructions below to make simple fried chicken.

1. Shake the spices, ground almonds, & herbs together in a plastic bag to combine.
2. Then add the chicken drumsticks, toss the bag, and rub the mixture all over the chicken. Using olive oil, coat the base of a baking dish.
3. Put the chicken drumsticks in the olive oil and bake for 25 minutes at 400°F in a preheated oven.
4. During cooking, flip the drumsticks 2 to 3 times to ensure that the entire coating is coated in olive oil.

Sizzler Chicken Wings

Cooking time: 20 minutes

Preparation time: 10 minutes

Servings: 4

Per serving: Calories 376, Total fat 29g, Protein 26g, Carbs 1g

Ingredients:

- 1 medium-sized onion, peeled & finely chopped
- 2 teaspoons of cumin seeds
- 12 skinless chicken wings
- 4 tablespoons of hot water
- 2 teaspoons of finely chopped garlic, peeled
- Salt & pepper to taste
- 2 teaspoons of ginger, peeled & finely chopped
- 1 finely chopped green chili
- 2 tablespoons of vegetable oil
- 2 teaspoons of soy sauce

Instructions:

Follow the instructions below to make sizzler chicken wings.

1. At 400°F, preheat the oven.
2. In a medium-sized skillet, heat the oil & sauté the onion in one tablespoon of it until golden brown, about four minutes.
3. Cook for another minute after adding the ginger and garlic.
4. Cook for another minute after adding the cumin seeds & chili, then remove the pan from the flame.
5. Toss the chicken wings with the soy sauce & onion mixture and mix completely for one minute.
6. Pour in the water and mix well before transferring the contents of the wok to an ovenproof dish.
7. Bake for around 20 minutes.
8. Allow for 5 minutes of resting time after cooking and enjoy!

Easy and Tasty Chicken Burgers

Cooking time: 15 minutes

Preparation time: 10 minutes

Servings: 4

Per serving: Calories 190, Total fat 8g, Protein 20.2g, Carbs 1g

Ingredients:

- 2 finely chopped medium onions
- 2 teaspoons of ground cumin
- 1/4 teaspoon of black pepper
- Tomato & lettuce to garnish
- 100 g of coarsely grated carrots
- 2 tablespoons of skimmed milk
- Salt to taste
- 2 teaspoons of finely chopped garlic
- 1/4 teaspoon of crushed dried Italian seasoning
- 400 g of chicken mince

Instructions:

Follow the instructions below to make easy and tasty chicken burgers.

1. In a mixing dish, combine the carrots, onions, garlic, cumin, black pepper, milk, Italian seasoning, and salt.
2. Mix in the chicken mince completely.
3. Form the mix into patties and cook for 4 minutes per side in a hot skillet. Serve with tomato & lettuce slices.

Dessert Recipes

Cheese and Cashew Flapjacks

Cooking time: 20 minutes

Preparation time: 10 minutes

Servings: 18

Per serving: Calories 141, Total fat 4g, Protein 5g, Carbs 8g

Ingredients:

- 100 g of chopped cashew
- 175 g of porridge oats
- 75 g of butter
- 1 medium-sized carrot
- 1 large lightly beaten free-range egg
- 175 g of grated medium cheddar cheese

Instructions:

Follow the instructions below to make cheese and cashew flapjacks.

1. At 380°F, preheat the oven. Grease an 8-inch-by-8-inch baking tray lightly. Melt the butter in a medium-sized saucepan on a low flame.
2. Remove the butter from the heat and stir in the cashews, oats, carrots, cheese, and egg. Fill the tin halfway with the ingredients & level it out with a spatula.
3. After that, bake the flapjacks for 20 minutes in a preheated oven.
4. Remove the baking sheet from the oven & place the flapjacks on a wire rack to cool. Cut the cake into 18 slices & enjoy!

Raspberry and Raw Apple Tart

Cooking time: 0 minutes

Preparation time: 15 minutes

Servings: 4

Per serving: Calories 617, Total fat 42g, Protein 14g, Carbs 24g

Ingredients:

- 100 g of pecan nuts
- 1/2 teaspoon of ground cinnamon
- 100 g of raw almonds
- A handful of raspberries
- 100 g of cashew nuts
- 100 g of apples, cut lengthways
- 6 soft dried dates

Instructions:

Follow the instructions below to make raspberry and raw apple tart.

1. In a blender, combine the pecan nuts, almonds, and cashew nuts & pulse until finely ground. Blend in the dates & cinnamon until they are thoroughly combined and evenly distributed.
2. Blend in four tablespoons of water to fully incorporate the ingredients.
3. Fill four loose-bottomed tartlet cases halfway with the mixture and push down. Serve with apple slices & raspberry on top.

Mouth-Watering Ricotta Cheesecake

Cooking time: 20 minutes

Preparation time: 10 minutes

Servings: 4

Per serving: Calories 318, Total fat 16g, Protein 17g, Carbs 23g

Ingredients:

- 1/2 tablespoon of agave nectar
- 100 g of fresh raspberries
- For the cheesecakes:
- 30 g of softened butter
- 1 tablespoon of agave nectar
- 100 g of digestive biscuits
- 3 eggs
- 1 teaspoon of vanilla essence
- 250 g of ricotta cheese

Instructions:

Follow the instructions below to make mouth-watering ricotta cheesecake.

1. For the raspberry coulis: Put 100g of raspberries in a blender with a little water and 1/2 a tablespoon of agave nectar to make a puree.
2. For the cheesecake: At 350°F, preheat the oven.
3. Grease 4 ramekin dishes or other small containers lightly.
4. Make crumbs out of the digestive biscuits. You can do this by smashing them with a rolling pin in a fully sealed bag.
5. After that, thoroughly combine the crumbs and butter. Alternatively, you may blitz the whole biscuits with butter in a food processor to speed up the process, but this will result in more dishes!

6. Separate the egg whites from the yolks by cracking the eggs & allowing the whites to drip into a dish without the yolks.
7. These must then be whisked for 4 minutes to achieve a silky texture. In a mixing dish, break up the ricotta.
8. Mix in the agave nectar, egg whites, and vanilla extract until all ingredients are fully combined. Fill the ramekin dishes halfway with the mixture.
9. 1Place the cheesecakes in the oven & bake for 20 minutes, or until brown. 1Add the raspberries & fruit coulis on top and enjoy!

Tasty Fruit Pizza

Cooking time: 0 minutes

Preparation time: 15 minutes

Servings: 8

Per serving: Calories 112, Total fat 9g, Protein 0.6g, Carbs 11g

Ingredients:

- 30 g of softened butter
- 200 g of strawberries
- 100 g of broken digestive biscuits
- Several mints leave for decoration
- 3 tablespoons of lemon curd

Instructions:

Follow the instructions below to make tasty fruit pizza.

1. Line a loose-bottomed 15-cm cake pan with greaseproof paper and lightly grease it with butter it's not the butter indicated in the ingredients.
2. Place the digestive biscuit pieces & butter in a food processor and pulse until the biscuits are finely crushed, and the butter is uniformly distributed.
3. Place the mixture in the prepared cake tin, flattening the buttery biscuit base into an equal layer using the back of a dessert spoon, and chill.
4. Pour the lemon curd atop the cooled base after one hour.
5. Place each strawberry on top of the lemon curd, cut it into four pieces. Before serving, garnish with mint leaves!
6. To avoid a soggy foundation, serve as quickly as it's ready.

Crunchy Oatcakes

Cooking time: 10 minutes

Preparation time: 10 minutes

Servings: 4

Per serving: Calories 70, Total fat 1g, Protein 2g, Carbs 18g

Ingredients:

- 50 g of plain flour
- 300 ml of warm water
- 150 g of fine Oatmeal
- 1 teaspoon of salt

Instructions:

Follow the instructions below to make crunchy oatcakes.

1. At 300°F, preheat the oven.
2. Mix the oatmeal, flour & salt in a mixing bowl. Slowly pour in the warm water.
3. Roll out the dough onto a floured surface & knead it until it is 1/4 inch thick. Cut into triangles & cook on a grill or in a pan.
4. Bake for around 3-4 minutes, or until crisp. Serve with a pat of butter.

Witches' Apples Dessert

Cooking time: 0 minutes

Preparation time: 15 minutes

Servings: 4

Per serving: Calories 95, Total fat 0.1g, Protein 5g, Carbs 17g

Ingredients:

- 100 ml of Greek yogurt
- Lollipop sticks
- 4 green apples around
- 133 g each Edible glitter
- Black food coloring

Instructions:

Follow the instructions below to make witches' apples dessert.

1. Insert a wooden lollipop stick into the middle of each apple after it has been rinsed. Combine the Greek yogurt & the black food coloring in a small-sized bowl.
2. Then, dip the bottom of each apple in the mixture, leaving the top green. Put the Witches' Apples on a baking tray upright.
3. Sprinkle edible glitter over each one and place in the freezer for 30 minutes or until the yogurt is set.

Crunchy Honey Oat Cookies

Cooking time: 10 minutes

Preparation time: 10 minutes

Servings: 15

Per serving: Calories 84, Total fat 6g, Protein 4g, Carbs 9g

Ingredients:

- 25 g of medium oatmeal
- 1 tablespoon of runny honey
- 60 ml of vegetable oil
- 1 tablespoon of pumpkin seeds
- 60 g of porridge oats
- 1 medium lightly beaten egg
- 60 g of Stevia
- 1 teaspoon of vanilla extract

Instructions:

Follow the instructions below to make crunchy honey oat cookies.

1. At 350°F, preheat the oven.
2. Using baking parchment, line an 8 x 8-inch baking tray.
3. In a large-sized mixing bowl, combine the oatmeal, porridge oats, Stevia, egg, honey, vanilla essence, oil, and pumpkin seeds.
4. Using a spatula, pour the mixture onto the baking tray & level it out. Bake the cookies for around 10 minutes or until golden brown.
5. Place them on a wire cooling rack once they've finished cooking.

Tasty Milk Pudding

Cooking time: 10 minutes

Preparation time: 20 minutes

Servings: 4

Per serving: Calories 318, Total fat 31g, Protein 3g, Carbs 8g

Ingredients:

- 220 g of double cream
- 4 teaspoons of vegetable oil
- 25 g of Stevia
- 1 teaspoon of agar-agar
- 75 g of buttermilk
- 250 ml of whole milk

For the syrup:

- 75 ml of boiling water
- 4 drops of rose water
- 75 g of Stevia
- Juice of a blood orange

Instructions:

Follow the instructions below to make tasty milk pudding.

1. In a large-sized mixing dish, combine the milk & buttermilk. Then, using the vegetable oil, grease four dariole molds & place them on a tray.
2. In a small-sized saucepan on a low flame, heat the double cream. Stir in the Stevia till it is completely dissolved.
3. After that, increase the flame to high & boil the cream for around 2 minutes. Combine the agar-agar and the cream mixture.

4. After that, pour the cream mixture over the milk and buttermilk in the dariole molds/ Place the mixture in the fridge to refrigerate overnight once it has cooled down.

TO MAKE THE SYRUP:

1. In a mixing bowl, combine the Stevia, blood orange juice, boiling water, & rose water.
2. Stir until all of the Stevia has dissolved.
3. Turn out the milk puddings by running a blunt knife all around the molds' & turning them out onto four plates.

Flavorful Pecan Pancakes

Cooking time: 10 minutes

Preparation time: 20 minutes

Servings: 4

Per serving: Calories 437, Total fat 27g, Protein 7g, Carbs 47g

Ingredients:

For the pancakes:

- 100 g of tapioca flour
- 400 ml of almond milk
- 100 g of rice flour
- 4 tablespoons of coconut oil
- 2 large-sized eggs

For the topping:

- 2 tablespoons of agave nectar
- 50 g of toasted pecans

Instructions:

Follow the instructions below to make flavorful pecan pancakes.

1. In a food processor, combine the rice flour, eggs, tapioca flour, and almond milk and process for 2 minutes.
2. Fill a jug halfway with the smooth batter.
3. Heat 1/2 a tablespoon of coconut oil for each pancake in a large nonstick frying pan. After that, pour 1/8 of the batter into the pan & swirl it around to form a full-size pancake. Cook for 2 minutes, or until golden around the sides of the pancake.
4. Turn the pancake around with a spatula and cook on the other side. Cooking the second side should only take a minute. Ascertain that both sides are golden. Then repeat the process with the remaining 8 pancakes.

5. Maintain the pancakes warm by wrapping them in foil and placing them in a low-temperature oven.
6. Layer 2 pancakes each dish onto a dish to plate up. Drizzle agave nectar over the pancakes and top with pecans.

Delicious Coconut Pannacotta

Cooking time: 10 minutes

Preparation time: 20 minutes

Servings: 2

Per serving: Calories 250, Total fat 38g, Protein 5g, Carbs 26g

Ingredients:

- 1 vanilla pod
- 4 tablespoons of pomegranate seeds
- 1 tin of coconut milk
- 1tablespoon of agar-agar flakes

Instructions:

Follow the instructions below to make delicious coconut pannacotta.

1. Place the coconut milk and agar agar in a separate pan & set aside.
2. By slicing open the vanilla bean lengthwise and removing the dark contents with the tip of a knife, put the vanilla with the coconut milk mixture.
3. Warm the mixture gently on medium flame while whisking continuously.
4. Continue to whisk until all of the agar-agar has dissolved. You'll need to boil the mixture for around 10 to15 minutes if you're using agar-agar flakes.
5. Remove the pan from the flame and divide the contents evenly among four serving bowls. Put them in the fridge to set, which should take around an hour.
6. Pomegranate seeds can be sprinkled on top of your food.

Tasty Ginger Snaps

Cooking time: 15 minutes

Preparation time: 10 minutes

Servings: 12

Per serving: Calories 106, Total fat 8g, Protein 4g, Carbs 7g

Ingredients:

- 2 teaspoons of pure vanilla extract
- 75 g of plain flour
- 1/2 tablespoon of minced ginger
- 50 g of soft pure vegetable margarine
- 1/2 teaspoon of grated nutmeg
- 50 g of Stevia
- 100 g of almond flour
- 2 tablespoons of finely chopped stem ginger
- 4 tablespoons of unsweetened soya milk
- 1/2 tablespoon of baking powder
- 2 teaspoons of ground cinnamon

Instructions:

Follow the instructions below to make tasty ginger snaps.

1. At 380°F, preheat the oven and prepare a baking pan with parchment paper.
2. In a large-sized mixing bowl, combine the vegetable margarine & Stevia and beat until light and creamy. It takes 3 to 4 minutes to do this task.
3. Add the vanilla extract & continue to beat.
4. Combine the plain flour, stem ginger, baking powder, nutmeg, ginger, cinnamon, and salt. To form a soft dough, add enough soya milk and roll the dough into Twelve balls.
5. Arrange the balls on the baking trays with some distance between them. Bake for 10 minutes, or until golden brown

until each ball has been flattened. Place the baked biscuits on a cooling rack for 5 minutes to cool.

Easy Homemade Jam

Cooking time: 25 minutes

Preparation time: 5 minutes

Servings: 4

Per serving: Calories 6, Total fat 0g, Protein 0.1g, Carbs 4g

Ingredients:

- 30 g of Triple Zero sweetener
- 1/2 teaspoon of Xanthan Gum
- 400 g of raspberries
- 40 drops of liquid vanilla Stevia

Instructions:

Follow the instructions below to make easy homemade jam.

1. In a saucepan, combine the Triple Zero Sweetener, raspberries, & vanilla Stevia and cook on low flame.
2. Slowly increase the flame while stirring continually.
3. Once the mixture has reached a boil, reduce the heat to low and continue to whisk regularly for 15 minutes.
4. Smash the raspberries using the back of a wooden spoon on the pan's side while mixing. Over the top of the mixture, stir in the Xanthan gum thoroughly.
5. Continue to simmer for 3 minutes after continuing to stir.
6. Turn off the flame, set the saucepan aside, cover it, and allow the jam to cool entirely.
7. The jam can be kept in the fridge in an airtight jar. The jam is prepared to use once it has been chilled.

Peachy Crumble

Cooking time: 25 minutes

Preparation time: 5 minutes

Servings: 6

Per serving: Calories 300, Total fat 25g, Protein 3g, Carbs 13g

Ingredients:
- 50 g of rolled oats
- 3 firm peaches
- 75 g of almond flour
- 100 g of soft pure vegetable margarine
- 50 g of flaked almonds
- 75 g of Stevia

Instructions:

Follow the instructions below to make a peachy crumble.

1. At 360°F, preheat the oven.
2. In a large-sized mixing dish, combine the rolled oats, almond flour, and Stevia to make the crumble.
3. Add the vegetable margarine & knead the mixture together using your fingertips until it resembles fine breadcrumbs.
4. Peel & slice the peaches, then layer them in the bottoms of 6 oven-safe ramekins. Spread the crumble over the peaches & distribute the flaked almonds on top.
5. Place the crumble in the oven and bake for around 25 minutes, or until golden brown.

Yummy Banana Brulee

Cooking time: 15 minutes

Preparation time: 10 minutes

Servings: 2

Per serving: Calories 234, Total fat 10g, Protein 6g, Carbs 35g

Ingredients:

- 1/2 tablespoon of lemon juice
- 4 tablespoons of Stevia
- 2 ripe medium-sized bananas, peeled & sliced
- 200 ml of Greek yogurt

Instructions:

Follow the instructions below to make a yummy banana Brulee.

1. Four banana slices are left aside & divided between 2 tiny ramekin dishes. Then, drizzle the lemon juice on the banana slices and place it in the refrigerator.
2. Meanwhile, in a small-sized saucepan on medium flame, combine the Stevia & 2 tablespoons of water.
3. Warm the combination until all of the sweetness has dissolved. After that, simmer the mix for 4 minutes, or until golden brown.
4. Spread the Stevia mixture over the yogurt in the ramekin dishes to serve. Finish with the remaining banana slices.

Dairy-Free Chocolate and Raspberry Mousse

Cooking time: 10 minutes

Preparation time: 15 minutes

Servings: 6

Per serving: Calories 169, Total fat 15g, Protein 3g, Carbs 21g

Ingredients:

- 100 g of soft silken tofu
- 50 g of coconut cream
- 100 g of dairy-free chocolate, at least 70% cocoa solids, roughly chopped
- 50 g of Stevia
- 150 g of raspberries
- 2 tablespoons of vanilla bean paste

Instructions:

Follow the instructions below to make dairy-free chocolate and raspberry mousse.

1. Place a medium-sized saucepan half-filled with boiling water on a medium flame.
2. Next, set a medium heatproof bowl on top, making sure the base is in contact with the water.
3. Place the roughly chopped chocolate in a mixing bowl and set it aside to melt, stirring occasionally.
4. After wringing excess water out from tofu with a clean tea towel, combine it with the Stevia & vanilla bean paste in a food processor.
5. Combine the melted chocolate & coconut cream. Pulse until the texture is smooth and velvety. Transfer to large-sized mixing dish.

6. Fold in the raspberries in a large-sized mixing dish, leaving a few for garnishing. Refrigerate for 30 minutes after dividing the mixture into 6 individual bowls.
7. Take it out of the fridge. Garnish with raspberries and a sprig of mint.

Yummy Fruit Frenzy

Cooking time: 10 minutes

Preparation time: 20 minutes

Servings: 4

Per serving: Calories 87, Total fat 0.9g, Protein 1g, Carbs 22g

Ingredients:

- 180 ml of semi-skimmed milk
- 100 g of raspberries
- 1 tablespoon of Stevia
- 100 g of canned peaches, drained
- 60 ml of water
- 1 1/2 tablespoons of agave nectar
- 100 g of canned pears, drained
- 1 tablespoon of corn flour

Instructions:

Follow the instructions below to make a yummy fruit frenzy.

1. In a small-sized bowl, add the raspberries.
2. Warm the water and stir in the Stevia till it dissolves and makes a syrup, then pour over the raspberries, making sure they are completely covered.
3. Put this in the refrigerator.
4. In a small dish, combine the corn flour, agave nectar, and 2 tablespoons of milk. Bring the remaining milk to a boil, then whisk in the corn flour mix to make a custard. Remove the pan from the flame and set it aside to cool.
5. Blend the pears & peaches until they are completely smooth.
6. Purée a few raspberries, reserving as many as you want to garnish with at the end. Set it aside. Stir in the thickened milk custard mixture to the pears & peaches thoroughly.

7. Fill a sundae/dessert dish halfway with the Stevia/raspberry combination. 1Top with the custard mixture and the raspberries that weren't puréed.
8. Allow between one-two hours to chill before serving.

Tasty Lemon Soufflé

Cooking time: 0 minutes

Preparation time: 20 minutes

Servings: 6

Per serving: Calories 258, Total fat 22g, Protein 6g, Carbs 1g

Ingredients:

- 3 tablespoons of Stevia
- 15 g of vegetarian gelatin
- 3 eggs
- 300 ml of double cream
- 2 large lemons rind and juice
- 4 tablespoons of hot water

Instructions:

Follow the instructions below to make a tasty lemon soufflé.

1. By shattering the egg & slowly tipping the contents from one side of the shell to the other, avoiding dropping the yolk, separate the yolks out of the egg whites. The egg whites should separate & drip through space do this over a bowl!
2. In a heatproof bowl, combine the lemon rind, egg yolks, Stevia, and lemon juice. Place the bowl over a pan of hot water to keep it warm.
3. With an electric whisk, whip the mixture till it hardens into a custard. This should take about 5 minutes to complete.
4. In 4 tablespoons of boiling water, dissolve the gelatin.
5. When the water/gelatin has reached room temperature, stir it into the lemon custard for 5 minutes.
6. To keep the texture, fold in the double cream with a spatula to spoon the mixture & put it over the top.

7. Stir the egg whites into the mixture after whisking them until they thicken and form stiff peaks. Place the mixture in 6 small ramekin cups in the refrigerator for 2 hours to set.

Tempting Chocolate Cake

Cooking time: 20 minutes

Preparation time: 10 minutes

Servings: 6

Per serving: Calories 225, Total fat 13g, Protein 5g, Carbs 22g

Ingredients:

For the chocolate sponge:

- 30 g of unsweetened cocoa powder
- 1/4 teaspoon of bicarbonate of soda
- 2 large-sized eggs
- 1 tablespoon of agave nectar
- 30 g of almond flour
- 150 g of full-fat ricotta cheese
- 60 ml of semi-skimmed milk
- 100 g of self-rising flour

For the cake topping:

- 60 ml of double cream
- Fresh berries for decoration
- 1 teaspoon of vanilla essence
- 1/2 teaspoon of agave nectar

Instructions:

Follow the instructions below to make a tempting chocolate cake.

1. At 380°F, preheat the oven.
2. To break up the yolks, crack the eggs & lightly whisk them in a separate dish. To soften the ricotta, beat it using a wooden spoon for about 3 minutes.
3. In a small bowl, combine the cocoa powder and a tablespoon of milk.

4. Combine the eggs, milk/ cocoa mixture, agave nectar, self-rising flour, remaining milk, bicarbonate of soda, & almond flour.
5. Line a 7-inch loose-bottomed cake tin with baking paper after lightly buttering it. Bake for around 20 minutes after pouring the batter into the pan.
6. Warm the vanilla essence, cream, & agave nectar in a small-sized saucepan on low flame, constantly stirring, to form the creamy topping.
7. Place the pan to the side and turn off the flame.
8. Spread the topping on top of the cake once the mixture has cooled. 1Enjoy the cake after you've decorated it with your favorite berries.

Yummy Kiwi Pavlova

Cooking time: 20 minutes

Preparation time: 10 minutes

Servings: 4

Per serving: Calories 142, Total fat 3g, Protein 7g, Carbs 18g

Ingredients:

- 25 g of blueberries
- 1/2 ripe mango
- 1/4 teaspoon of cream of tartar
- 4 large-sized free-range eggs whites
- A pinch of salt
- 25 g of Triple Zero sweetener
- 50 g of strawberries
- 25 g of raspberries
- 4 kiwi fruit
- 1 teaspoon of vanilla essence

Instructions:

Follow the instructions below to make a yummy kiwi pavlova.

1. At 450°F, preheat the oven.
2. Grease a baking tray with butter after lining it with grease-proof paper.
3. By shattering the eggs' shells and pouring the whites into a dish while holding the yolks back, separate the eggs.
4. Beat the egg whites with an electric whisk until stiff, then season with a touch of salt & cream of tartar.
5. Fold the vanilla extract & Triple Zero sweetener into the egg whites using a spatula. This will guarantee that the ingredients are fully combined without the eggs losing their firm quality.

6. Spoon the precise amount of mixture for each meringue nest onto the baking tray that has been prepared. For the fruit topping, make a little dip in each one.
7. Bake for around 20 minutes. After that, put it aside to cool down.
8. Enjoy the raspberries, mango slices, kiwi, and strawberries on top of the meringue nests!

Tasty Almond Cupcakes

Cooking time: 15 minutes

Preparation time: 10 minutes

Servings: 12

Per serving: Calories 113, Total fat 7g, Protein 1g, Carbs 1g

Ingredients:

- 2 teaspoons of baking powder
- 80 ml of water
- Pinch of salt
- 200 g of almond flour
- 100 g of melted butter
- 80 ml of liquid artificial sweetener
- 4 eggs

Instructions:

Follow the instructions below to make tasty almond cupcakes.

1. At 350°F, preheat the oven.
2. Cupcake liners should be used to line a baking tray.
3. In a large-sized mixing dish, sift together the baking powder & sweetener. Make sure there are no lumps in the almond flour by sifting it in.
4. In a separate jug beat the eggs and slowly add the butter & water.
5. Pour the egg mixture into the dry flour mixture quickly, steady stream, stirring constantly. If the mixture appears to be curdling, simply add a bit more almond flour.
6. Fill the cupcake liners halfway with the batter and bake for 15 minutes in a hot oven. Allow time for the dish to cool prior to serving.

Conclusion

Diabetes mellitus is on the rise, and if not managed properly, it can lead to life- threatening complications. Because of the personal and financial costs associated with diabetes care, there are numerous hurdles in successfully treating diabetes mellitus. Its long-term implications result in a great deal of human misery and financial losses. Comprehensive diabetes care, on the other hand, can help to delay the onset of problems, improve quality of life, and reduce healthcare costs.

Insulin is used to treat diabetes mellitus in all forms. Diet, exercise, & diabetes education, on the other hand, remain critical components of diabetic treatment. Obesity should be forcefully addressed, and lifestyle improvements should be prioritized.